# A Society Clown

George Grossmith

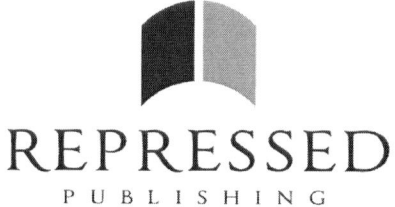
REPRESSED
PUBLISHING

© 2013 Repressed Publishing LLC All rights reserved.

ISBN: 978-1-4622-8808-3

Printed in the United States of America
Repressed Publishing LLC
Provo, Utah

www.repressedpublishing.com

*Copyright. Entered at Stationers' Hall*

# A SOCIETY CLOWN

### REMINISCENCES

BY

## GEORGE GROSSMITH

**Arrowsmith's Bristol Library**
Vol. XXXI

BRISTOL
J. W. ARROWSMITH, 11 QUAY STREET
LONDON
SIMPKIN, MARSHALL & Co., 4 STATIONERS' HALL COURT
1888

## Dedicated

TO ONE

WHO BESIDES BEING MY WIFE

HAS ALSO BEEN MY TRUEST FRIEND AND

MY BEST ADVISER.

# CONTENTS.

| Chap. | | Page |
|---|---|---|
| I. | EXPLANATORY | 1 |
| II. | EARLY RECOLLECTIONS | 5 |
| III. | AT BOW STREET POLICE COURT | 19 |
| IV. | FROM AMATEUR TO PROFESSIONAL | 36 |
| V. | IN THE PROVINCES | 60 |
| VI. | GILBERT AND SULLIVAN | 91 |
| VII. | A SOCIETY CLOWN | 126 |
| VIII. | A VERY SNOBBISH CHAPTER | 155 |

# A SOCIETY CLOWN.

## CHAPTER I.

### Explanatory.

"You've no idea what a poor opinion I have of myself, and how little I deserve it."—*Ruddigore.*

IT was one dark, dank, dreary, dismal night in February, 1888 (I believe that is the way to commence a book, no matter what the subject be), when the present writer might have been seen standing, with other gentlemen, in a sombre dining-room brilliantly illuminated with one ceiling-lamp buried in a deep red shade. We were standing round the dining-room table, each with a dinner-napkin in the left hand; while the right hand was occupied in moving back chairs, to permit of the departure of the ladies for the drawing-room. I could not help thinking that, as they filed off, the ladies looked like queens; while we (especially with the aid of the serviettes) looked like waiters. The gentlemen drew their chairs round the host, and wine was languidly passed round. A tall gentleman, with a heavy beard, to whom I had not been introduced, approached me, and sat by my side. He passed me the spirit-lamp, for which I thanked him while lighting my cigarette. He then commenced a conversation in earnest.

"Did you see that Mr. —— is writing his reminiscences?"

"Yes."

"Don't you think it rather a pity that he should do so?"

"Why a pity?" I asked in reply to his question.

"Well, I always think the moment a man begins to write his reminiscences he is bound, more or less, to make an ass of himself."

"In what way?" I asked.

"In the first place, he is hampered by having to be so egotistical. He must talk about himself, which is never a nice thing to do. He cannot very well tell stories in his own favour; and if he tells them against himself, he affects humility: if he talks about his distinguished acquaintances, he becomes a snob; in short, I can only repeat my former observation, that he is bound to make an ass of himself."

For a moment or two I did not know what to say, for my conscience smote me. At last I said:

"I am very pleased to hear your candid, and certainly unbiassed, opinion; for I have just accepted an offer from Mr. Arrowsmith to do a shilling book of my own reminiscences for the Bristol Library Series."

My friend did not know what to say for a moment. His conscience evidently smote him. At last he remarked:

"I fear I have said one of those things that are best left unsaid."

"I'm glad you said it," I replied. "You have rather opened my eyes. It will be necessary for me to explain that I cannot very well back out of my agreement with Mr. Arrowsmith, although, candidly speaking, I have no desire to do so; and I shall certainly have to apologise to the reading public for making an ass of myself."

I have thought over the above conversation many a time since, and have concluded that I could not do better than commence this little book with it.

I have taken my own professional career, and used it as a peg whereon to hang my stories. I have chosen the title because I think it will look well on the bookstalls. It is by no means intended as a sneer at my calling. To clown properly is a very difficult art, and I am never so happy as when I am making people laugh. I am unfeignedly proud of my profession, on and off the stage. I have clowned amongst all sorts of people, and in all sorts of places. On the stage I play the fool of others' creation, and at the piano I play the simple fool of my own.

The late John Parry, whom I took as my model, was marvellous at amusing. His satire was worthy of Dickens or Thackeray. Though possessed of a small voice, few people could sing better, and certainly few could play the piano better than he. His was an "excellent fooling" that many have envied, many imitated, and none surpassed.

My first desire in producing the following sketches of my life is to benefit others, by making an hour pass pleasantly in the library or in a railway carriage. My second desire, which goes without saying, is to benefit my publisher and myself.

Like all clowns, I have had my serious side of life—I have experienced many small troubles and some sorrows ; but I shall not dwell on them, but merely reproduce some short notes— (having been a reporter, I may say *shorthand notes*)—of incidents which have amused me, and which I hope will equally entertain my readers. The majority I have had permission to publish, and the others I do not expect will be recognised. It would grieve me very much if I thought I had offended anyone.

Society has been exceedingly kind to its clown, and the clown is deeply grateful. My only ambition is, that someone in the dim future may speak half as kindly of me as Hamlet, Prince of Denmark, spoke of the Society Clown of his period.

## CHAPTER II.

### Early Recollections.

*"A many years ago, when I was young and charming."*
*H.M.S. Pinafore.*

AS I was born in December, 1847, I was not five years old when I was taken to a house at the corner of Wellington Street, Strand, to see the funeral procession of the Duke of Wellington. And I remember it as distinctly as if it had been yesterday. The crowd, the soldiers, and the magnificent funeral car, are still strongly engraven on my memory. That was the most important of my earlier recollections.

The next recollection of great importance was my having fallen desperately in love with a Miss Field, at a day-school near Bloomsbury, to which I was taken at five years of age, and which was kept by a Miss Adams. It was an academy for young (extremely young) ladies and gentlemen. It was only natural that I should desire to make my *fiancée* a suitable gift as a token of our engagement; so I presented her with a set of large gold shirt-studs, which I annexed from my father's dressing-table. The mother of my adored one, without having the courtesy to consult her daughter or myself, took the gift from the former, and returned it to the father of the latter. My parent explained to me the etiquette with regard to acts of alienation in a sweet, simple, and comprehensive manner worthy of Dr. Watts, and extracted from me a promise that in future I would discard that humour which had prompted me to generously dispose of other people's property. That promise I have faithfully kept.

As a reward for my future good intentions, he handed me a sovereign, with injunctions not to spend it. I must confess I could not see his object. A few days afterwards I began to be suspicious of his sovereign. There was some writing on one side, which I was not yet intelligent enough to decipher; but on the other, instead of the pretty head of our Most Gracious Majesty, there was an impression of a hat. I was much worried and concerned about that hat. I perfectly remember going to my parents and saying, "I would rather have a sovereign without a hat on." I also remember with what continued roars of laughter my request was met. I have the sovereign to this day. It is a brass disc, the exact size of a sovereign, advertising the Gibus opera hat.

About 1855 I was sent to a preparatory school kept by the Misses Hay, at Massingham House, Haverstock Hill. I was a boarder, and it was there I first began to play the fool. I invented several shadow pantomimes, and acted in them. As no dialogue was required, I can say nothing of my literary ability. On one occasion, when my mother visited me, she asked how I was getting on with my lessons. Miss Eliza Hay (from whom I had a letter last May) said, "He gets on very well with his music, but I am afraid he will one day be a clown."

I mention this because, about fifteen years

afterwards, my father met her, and informed her that I had made my appearance at the Polytechnic Institution as a professional entertainer, and she replied, "Ah! I always said he would be a clown." This is not repeated with any unkind intention, for the remarks were made by Miss Hay in a pure spirit of chaff. She was very kind to me, gave me lessons in elocution, and taught me pieces of poetry to recite. She used to write poetry herself.

Her sister, Miss Isabelle, taught me the piano; and, of course, I learned the "Prière d'une Vierge" and "Les Cloches de Monastère," and the "Duet in D" by Diabelli, to say nothing of Czerny's 101 exercises, all of which I used to play tolerably well at the age of nine and ten. Miss Isabelle also sang very nicely; and as I was very fond of music, I became a favourite pupil, and was taken by her to local concerts, where she sang for charities. Of course, I fell over head and ears in love with her.

The school was kept by three sisters, and the elder was a handsome lady with grey hair. She was an immense favourite with the boys. I have never forgotten her kindness in occasionally permitting me to fire off a brass cannon with real gunpowder in the kitchen. That was the sort of extension of license that a boy appreciated.

In 1856 I witnessed, from the lower part of Primrose Hill, the fireworks in celebration of peace with Russia. The final sight was wonderful, and greatly impressed me. At a given period, thousands of rockets were fired from the Hill and all the parks.

I was sometimes taken to the theatre, and have a faint recollection of Wright at the Adelphi, and a more distinct one of T. P. Cooke in *Black-eyed Susan*. I was afterwards introduced to him at Margate, and surprised to find he looked so old—which he certainly did not on the stage. It was in this year, I think, that I was taken to see the ruins of Covent Garden Theatre. It was the day after the fire, and smoke was still ascending in columns. I described this with characteristic exaggeration, and became a temporary hero at the school of the Misses Hay.

In 1857 my father took the little house now known as 36 Haverstock Hill. It was then known as 9 Powis Place, and was called Manor Lodge. My school was only a few doors off, and so I became a day scholar. I remained at this preparatory school until I was nearly twelve, and I can safely say I was very happy in those days. I do not mean to infer that I am not happy now. Fortunately, I am of an extremely happy disposition, and I so thoroughly enjoy the bright side of life that its shadows sink into insignificance.

Amongst my school-fellows at the Misses Hay's was Dr. Arthur W. Orwin, of the Throat and Ear Hospital, Gray's Inn Road.

In 1860 there was a Pugilistic Fever in England. Tom Sayers fought J. C. Heenan, the Benicia Boy. The fever was very virulent. It attacked Peers, Commons, Bishops, Actors, Soldiers, Sailors, Tinkers and Tailors. It attacked *The Times*, and all the daily, evening, weekly, monthly, quarterly, and yearly periodicals. Is it to be wondered at, that it attacked also the school of the Misses Hay? Tom Sayers, with his big dog, had been pointed out to me; so had Heenan and Tom King.

I was surreptitiously, and most certainly without the knowledge of my parents, taken by one of the servants at home to the house of Mr. Ben Caunt, who shook hands with me and showed me the room where boxing matches took place. I was then taken across the road, and this boy of twelve years and a few months was presented to Nat Langham. I was accordingly seized with the fever very badly. On the inside of my leather belt I sketched little panels of my imagined victories, and issued a challenge to fight anyone for the championship of the school—the victor to hold the leather belt. As I had shaken hands with Ben Caunt and Nat Langham, the boys were rather afraid of me. Orwin, however, accepted the challenge, threw his castor into the ring, and we fought for twenty minutes or half an hour: it seemed years to me. In the end I was undoubtedly defeated. One generally hears that corruption is the aim and end of all fights. I knew nothing of such practices then, and so cannot explain what induced me to offer Orwin twopence to admit that I was the conqueror, or what persuaded him to accept the sum and condition.

After leaving the preparatory school, I was sent to the North London Collegiate School, then under the headmastership of Dr. Williams. I wore a "mortar-board," and walked to and from the school with E. H. Dickens, who was a nephew of Charles Dickens, and who, living close to my home, became (and still is) a great friend of mine. The chief delight of the little home on Haverstock Hill was the garden at the back. It was much prettier than the modern suburban garden. There used to be nine apple trees and two pear trees. As time wore on, a couple of the trees wore out. My mother used to send the apples away to friends in basketsful. My brother Weedon and I generally partook of this fruit when it had grown to the size of a chestnut, and was particularly hard and green. We much preferred it to the mature apple. In this respect I think we resembled most boys.

When the bicycle came in vogue, a few years after, we three boys procured one each. (I include my father as one of the boys. It was his own desire, as well as his nature, to be one of us, and I often think many fathers would find it to their advantage if they followed his example). I possessed, what was considered then, a very high bicycle, the front wheel being 36 inches high. I got one for my brother, cheap, at an auction-room near Covent Garden. Being considered the champion rider of the three, I was sent to bid for the steed, and ride it home in style. I succeeded in the former, but not in the latter. Before an admiring crowd of Covent Garden loungers, loafers, porters, fruiterers, flower-girls and policemen, I leapt on to the saddle, and immediately broke the back of the spring, which had evidently been carefully made of cast-iron. My intention was that the bicycle should carry me home, but we reversed the order of things.

The steed used by my father stood about two and a half feet from the ground, and had iron wheels.

He himself was only a little over five feet, and was much—very much—inclined to *embonpoint*.

In the winter, the garden-path at Manor Lodge was a fine field for practice. I forget how many laps went to the mile; all I remember is, that three miles about did for Weedon and myself, and half a mile did for the Guv'nor—that is, if he had not done for himself before then. I never recollect anything so funny as seeing him trundling round the garden. It somewhat resembled a diminutive edition of the modern road engine. We heard him in the house distinctly—loud as he approached the house, the noise becoming less as he reached the bottom of the garden. Sometimes the noise would suddenly cease. Ha! We in the house knew instinctively what had happened, and rushed to the windows to look out. Yes; there he was, in the thick of the gooseberry bushes. Not on the bicycle—oh dear, no! Under it, most decidedly under it. Sometimes on these occasions we would push up the windows, and, in conjunction with our dear mother, greet him with a loud guffaw. Sometimes we would preserve a strict silence and listen. We heard him wheel the vehicle back, place it against the lattice-work of the verandah, open the door, and, as usual, call for me.

"George—George!"

"Here I am. What is it?"

"Oh, I say, George, have you got a piece of sticking-plaister?"

He always appealed to me for this article, knowing that I was in possession of a few quires of court plaister; for it was at this period I had commenced to shave.

In summer my mother would not permit the

bicycles in the garden because of the flowers, in which she took pride. In the earlier days at Manor Lodge the garden was a mass of roses. As the demon builders began to surround the locality, so the roses began to die, and blight began to kill the apple-trees.

Still, the garden always looked pretty, especially in the summer and autumn. Then we three boys went in for amateur photography. The fad was started by me, and I was the principal operator. A "dark room" was erected against the wall near the house, and the front was manufactured out of the folding doors which had formerly separated the dining-room from the drawing-room. An amateur photographer was a scarcity in those days. The clean and easy dry-plate process was not then in use. We first had to clean the plain glass plate, which, in my case, was never successfully accomplished; then to coat it with collodion, which, if it did not run off the plate up the sleeve, generally "set" in diagonal streaks. Then it had to be placed in the wet silver bath, an extremely sensitive concoction, which got out of order without the slightest provocation. After its exposure in the camera (by-the-by, I generally forgot to pull up the shutter, or, if I remembered that, discovered when I went to uncover the lens that its cap was already off), this plate was subjected to a development which was original in its vagaries.

If the figures on the plate were indistinct, it was more than could be said of the spots and patches which appeared vividly on the fingers and clothes. Still, I was devoted to the occupation while in my teens, and would photograph all day long, anybody or anything. The family sat or stood to me a dozen times a day. The dogs used to sneak into the house and hide in the coal cellar the moment they saw me bring out the camera. The tradesmen and servants were all taken. All my father's friends, and they were numerous and good-natured, were seized and carried into the garden to be taken on glass; for I generally took "positives," which were finished off then and there and put into little brass frames, like the sixpenny and shilling portraits (eighteenpence if a bit of jewellery is painted in with gold) one sees displayed in the Euston Road and elsewhere.

I have taken Toole scores of times, H. J. Byron, J. Billington, Andrew Halliday, and many more: in fact, the last-named wrote an article in *All the Year Round* called "Precocious Boys," in which he described my brother and myself photographing him in a back-garden. I hope the reader will not think I am boasting, but I can solemnly declare that I do not believe any photographer, professional or amateur, ever succeeded in turning out so many deplorable failures as I did.

I attach rather an interesting programme of a juvenile—followed by a grown-up—party at Manor Lodge:

Haverstock Hill, April 1st, 1864.
*With Master George and Walter Grossmith's Compliments.*

PROGRAMME.

7 o'clock.—General Gathering of the Company (Limited).
The first arrival will please to make itself as comfortable as possible.

7.30.—Music and Conversation. The latter may be
varied by an occasional allusion to the day of
the month—a practical joke being the
"touch of nature" that makes
everybody *touchy*.

8 o'clock.—Quadrille and Polka. After which, Mrs.
Martha Brown (from the Egyptian Hall) will
describe her "Trip to Brighton and
back."

9 o'clock.—Quadrille and Waltz.

A few young gents in their teens, inspired by
the Tercent-*e*-nary (see Hepworth Dixon or any other
dixon-ary), will recite a passage from—and a
very long way from—HAMLET.

9.30.—Quadrille. Polka. Spanish Dance.

10 o'clock.—THE JUVENILE SPREAD. Children under
20 not admitted.

10.30.—The author of "*Underground* London" will
demon-strate his well-known connection with
the arch-enemy. (Beware of your
pockets.)

11.—Dancing, Comic Singing, etc.

12 to 1.—Arrival of the Professionals from the Royal
Adelphi, Olympic, St. James's, and Princess's
Theatres, retained at an enormous cost
for this night only—or rather
morning.

BANQUET OF THE ELDERS IN THE CULINARY CAVERNS
OF THE REGIONS BELOW.

Resumption of the fun. Paul's return a *great* go. Curious
analysis of the Brothers Webb, to ascertain
which is which.
Mr. Toole will oblige, etc.

Any attempt to define the order or duration of the proceedings from this point being obviously absurd, it will suffice to state that the Sun rises at 5.30.

The twenty minutes' burlesque on *Hamlet*
was written expressly for us by my father. It
was received so well that we afterwards did it

at the residences of Mr. Toole and John Hollingshead to "grown-up" parties, of which we were very proud. I played Hamlet, my brother played Ophelia and the Gravedigger, and the remainder of the characters were assumed by schoolfellows at the North London Collegiate School, who were, singularly enough, distantly connected with the stage. They were Pierre Leclercq, the brother of Carlotta Leclercq; Claude Addison, brother of the Misses Fanny and Carlotta Addison; B. Terry, brother of Ellen Terry, who, with her sister Kate (Mrs. Arthur Lewis), visited Manor Lodge several times. The part of the Queen was played by T. Bolton, who afterwards went on the stage and became a prominent member of Mr. Wilson Barrett's provincial companies. Many actors and literary men and women came in late at this party.

I knew very little of Society (with a big S) in those days, but had the honour, under the parental roof, of meeting and making friends, while a young man, of such people as Henry Irving, Toole, J. Clarke (Little Clarke, as he was called), H. J. Byron, John Oxenford, Kate and Ellen Terry, Madame Celeste, Miss Woolgar, Andrew Halliday, Artemus Ward, Chas. Wyndham, the brothers Brough, Luke Fildes, R.A., Joseph Hatton, Dillon Croker, J. Prowse, Fred Barnard, Mrs. Eiloart, Eliza Winstanley, Emma Stanley (the entertainer), W. S. Woodin, Arthur Sketchley, Tom Hood the younger, T. W. Robertson, Miss Furtardo, Paul Bedford.

For eight or nine months in the year we did not see much of the master of the house, for he was away lecturing; but we always welcomed his return home, generally on Saturdays. In the summer he had more leisure; he was brimful of humour, and there were few people so good at repartee.

When he was "put out," there was no mistaking it. He would then *speak* without thinking; but he never *wrote* without thinking. What a deal of trouble would be saved in this world if people would only delay answering an annoying letter for twenty-four hours!

Some of my father's replies were very amusing, I remember. I happened to come across a copy of one recently. I must first explain that my mother was passionately fond of animals, and had a strong tendency to overfeed them. In the next garden to ours a dog was chained close to the adjoining wall, and I have no doubt whatever that every remnant of food was dropped over for his special delight. The next-door neighbour wrote a sharp remonstrance, and complained that his dog was getting too fat in consequence of its being overfed. My father wrote the following characteristic reply:

"9 Powis Place,
"*December* 18*th*, 1870.

"Dear Sir,—I am very sorry my people have annoyed you by giving food to your dog.

"Mrs. Grossmith happens to be very fond of dogs. I think she prefers them to human beings, and she has a notion that it is very cruel to keep one chained up eternally; and possibly this want of exercise may have more to do with its getting fat than the occasional extra feeding to which you refer, and which comes of weak womanly sympathy with misfortune—just as our booby philanthropists, after contributing nearly half a million for the relief of the sick and wounded, received nothing but kicks and growls from the ruffianly savages in return.

"Seriously, however, you have a perfect right to complain, and I have given orders which I hope will be obeyed. I am very seldom in London myself, and cannot boast of having much control over my household when I am; but I think I may rely on your wishes being implicitly regarded.

"I almost wonder that it has not occurred to you to put the dog on the other side of the garden, out of their reach; but I trust there will be no occasion for this now.

"Yours faithfully,
"GEO. GROSSMITH.
—— Esq."

The next-door neighbour was amused with this letter, having taken it in its proper spirit, and became a visitor to the house. "All's well that ends well."

In accordance with its usual custom, time rolled on. I began to exhibit a taste for painting, and my brother Weedon for acting. These professions we subsequently reversed. Weedon (his full name is Walter Weedon Grossmith) left the North London Collegiate School to go to school nearer home; viz., Mr. Simpson's, in Belsize Park. Eventually I left the N.L.C.S to go to Bow Street, with the ultimate intention of entering for the bar; and Weedon, after leaving school, went to the West London School of Art in Portland Street, also to the Slade School at the London University, and eventually he passed the requisite examination that admitted him to the Royal Academy Schools.

I have endeavoured to make this little sketch of my old home as brief as possible, and will conclude this chapter with an incident that ultimately happened to be of considerable importance to me:

At a certain juvenile party, while still in jackets and turned-down collars, I met and became enamoured of a little maiden in a short frock and sash.

She flattered me by approving of my comic songs; and I was immensely struck with her power of conversation, which was unusual for one so young. I ascertained that her name was Emmeline Rosa Noyce, and that she was the only daughter of Doctor Noyce, whose practice was in the neighbourhood. We danced every dance together; but the Fates decreed that we should not meet again for another three or four years. We *did* meet—in a crowd, and again danced *nearly* every dance together; for, strange to say, she understood my step.

All this was simply a beginning to a very happy end: and I can say with truth that the wisest step I ever took in the whole course of my life was when, on the 14th May, 1873, I made my juvenile sweetheart my wife—with her consent, of course,—and, thank God, I have never had reason to regret it for a single second.

## CHAPTER III.

### At Bow Street Police Court.

*"Take down our sentence as we speak it."—Iolanthe.*

FOR a period of twenty years I had the distinguished honour of being decidedly "well known to the police." When I was between seventeen and eighteen years of age, and still at the North London Collegiate School, I received instructions from my father, who was just starting for Liverpool, that as Mr. Courtenay was ill I must go and "do" Bow Street. Mr. John Kelly Courtenay used to do all the reporting at Bow Street Police Court during my father's absence on his lecturing tours. I had learned shorthand (the Lewisian system, I believe it was called) some two or three years previously.

Off I marched to Bow Street with the greatest *sang-froid* to report a case, at which in after years I should certainly have shied. It was a most important bank fraud, and meant enormous complications in figures. Mr. Burnaby, then chief clerk, was kind enough to let me correct my figures from the depositions which had been taken by him; Sir Thomas Henry repeated to me the gist of his remarks on remanding the case, and the result was I turned out a report on manifold for all the evening and morning papers, and the usual special report for *The Times*—in this instance over a column long—with which my father was delighted.

I received a most encouraging letter from him after a few days' interval. The interval was merely to give time for the arrival of any complaint from the papers. Editors are not in the habit of sending letters of congratulation, only of complaint. No complaint arrived, however, and my only disappointment was the complete absence of important and interesting cases.

At last another opportunity arrived which enabled me to distinguish myself. I wish it had not. A poor woman was charged with purloining a shirt which was hanging outside a cheap hosier's in Clare Market somewhere. It was a windy day, and the end of the shirt was apparently flapping round the corner of the shop; so the prisoner, unable to resist temptation, filched it after the manner of a clown in a pantomime. Inspired by the punning humour of Tom Hood, I parodied one of his poems for the heading of my police report. The heading was "The Tale of a Shirt." This had a most undesired effect. The serious papers wrote to complain of the flippancy of the title; the refined papers of its vulgarity; while the vulgar papers inserted the title, which they emphasised by printing the word "tale" in italic.

This caused sarcastic paragraphs to appear in other papers directed against my father, who, of course, was the responsible reporter, and who, consequently, wrote me a second letter anent my talents for reporting which differed widely from the first.

Fortunately for all parties, Mr. Courtenay got well and returned to his post, and in 1866 it was decided I should thoroughly learn the business from him, so as to have some remunerative occupation while studying, and eventually following, the profession of the bar. Circumstances, however, ultimately prevented me from doing either. There are several, if not many, barrister-reporters in London; I know my friend Mr. E. T. Besley was one, and so were Mr. Finlayson and Mr. Corrie Grant, and I could mention three or four others.

My parent, with an eye to business, pointed out the absolute advantage that would arise from my being able to support myself by the press during the years I should, in all probability, be waiting for the arrival of a brief. His suggestion was adopted, and for the next three years I stuck entirely to the work, assisting Mr. Courtenay, who, in his turn, often assisted me in revising little occasional articles or verses which I wrote for humorous periodicals, &c., some of which were inserted to my great delight. He used to write prologues for amateur performances in which I took part, and at which he was always present. He was very kind to me, and I became very much attached to him, feeling great grief when he died in October, 1869.

The whole of the work then fell upon my shoulders during the absence of Grossmith, senior; and very hard work it was sometimes. When there was no work to do,—that is, nothing of consequence to report,—then the life of a reporter resembled that of a superior loafer—at least, that was my feeling. A reporter is not considered a sufficiently important person to be allotted a room for his own use. Sir Thomas Henry promised that the gentlemen of the press should have a room to themselves in the new Court, but he was unable to carry his promise out, as he died soon afterwards.

Therefore, when nothing was going on, the reporter became a kind of Micawber hanging about waiting for something to turn up. I used to sit in Court and write the opening chapters of three-volume novels which were never published, or extra verses to comic songs which were never sung.

When tired of this I used to loiter about the passages, or sit in the usher's room in company with solicitors, solicitors' clerks, witnesses with and without babies, detectives, defendants, and equally interesting people. Sometimes I meandered into the gaoler's room and gazed at the police and the prisoners. Sometimes I would go out to lunch and take three or four hours over it, and on returning find a most important murder case had been disposed of in my absence.

On one occasion I returned and found Mr. John Brown giving evidence in a charge against a lad for an attempt upon the life of our Most Gracious Majesty. However, I have managed to write a case just as well when I have not been present as when I have. The Court was a miserable one for sound, but the clerk was close to the witnesses and could hear them; so that his notes, which with courtesy I was permitted to copy, were, at all events, most reliable.

It must not be inferred from my absence that I was not interested in the work. On the contrary, there was so much variety in the important cases that one could not be otherwise than interested: but one never knew when they were coming on. But people of all classes would come day after day, and sit out (especially on a Monday morning) dozens of simple charges of drunk and disorderly, or of fighting and disturbing. This I could not quite understand. The days on which Mr. Flowers sat were certainly the most amusing, and consequently selected by the visitors. Mr. Irving, Mr. Toole, and the late George Belmore have often in bygone days sat by my side watching the more important cases.

Sometimes the monotony of the proceedings would be varied by my seeing one of my own acquaintances in the dock. Then an awkward question of etiquette arose. The dock joined the reporters' box. Now ought I to have shaken hands with him? As a matter of fact I never did, but I do not see why I should not have done so. However, I thought it best to follow the footsteps of the magistrates—they did not shake hands with their friends when charged.

I have heard of an instance of a metropolitan police magistrate who, upon recognising an old friend in dock, ordered him immediately to be accommodated with a seat on the bench and declined to hear the charge of embezzlement that was to have been preferred against him. Soon he was no more a magistrate, and subsequently was "no more" in the term's other sense.

The most disagreeable case of recognising a friend in the dock that I ever experienced was some years after, when I was combining the professions of journalist and entertainer. I accepted an engagement at Margate to give a couple of sketches nightly at the Hall-by-the-Sea, which was then under the management of the late E. P. Hingston, who had been formerly the manager of Artemus Ward's lecture at the Egyptian Hall in 1866. [By-the-by, the only other humorist who took part in the concert was J. Hatton, the composer and author of "To Anthea," who used to take his seat at the piano and sing his song, "Old Simon the Cellarer" and "The Merry Little Fat Grey Man," his resemblance to the latter being somewhat pronounced. He used to reside at Margate, and was an immense favourite.]

One evening I was introduced to a young gentleman of good manners and appearance, who begged I would sup with him. I did. We afterwards became rather intimate and I lunched with him. Like most small stars, I was surrounded by a lot of satellites. They were all eventually introduced to my new acquaintance, who seemed to have plenty of time and money to spare, and who was the essence of hospitality. As my engagement was terminating he gave us all a parting banquet at one of the principal hotels. Some old friend of mine had advised me particularly not to go. What reason he gave I do not remember, but I fancy it was that the young fellow had not paid some bill. However, I did not go, but heard there was much to eat, more to drink, and any amount of conviviality.

It was one of those parties where everybody talked, nobody listened, nobody cared, and every man's health was proposed by somebody else: the health of the host, I believe, was proposed about half a dozen times.

I returned to Bow Street, and a few days after this poor fellow, who turned out to be a clerk in a warehouse in Southampton Street, Strand, at about 35s. a week, was placed in the dock on a charge of robbing his employer. He was committed for trial and ultimately convicted; but in consequence of his previous good character and the kindness of his employer in not wishing to press the charge, the sentence was one of months when it might have been years.

I spent part of the spare time, in my earlier days at Bow Street, in editing a paper called *Ourselves at Home*. It was published by a printer for me, and consisted of eight pages, a little larger than the Bristol Library Series, with very little matter—much spacing out and very big type. The cost was ten shillings a week, for which we had fifty or a hundred copies.

Two of my friends contributed each two shillings and sixpence a week towards the expense, with the privilege of inserting articles. The contribution of their specie was more valuable than that of their brains; but as their contributions were not so bad as mine, no complaint was made. The periodical terminated after thirteen numbers, because our friends could not be induced to read it, much less buy it. It died a natural death on March 8th, 1867.

At this time the chief magistrate was Sir Thomas Henry, the other two being the kind and genial Mr. Flowers, who died only a few years ago, and Mr. James Vaughan, who still sits in the new Court. The old Court was adjacent to the Floral Hall, Covent Garden.

Having sat in that Court so many years, it seemed odd to me to pay it a visit under such different circumstances. Last summer (1887) I was advised to go to Mr. Stinchcombe, the theatrical costumier, on some little matter. I entered the front door of the old familiar Police Court. Instead of the idle, motley crowd one was accustomed to see blocking up the passages, there were rows of shelves with carefully-packed costumes.

In the Court, the dock, attorneys' table, barristers' bench, my old reporters' box, every partition in fact, had been swept away to make room for shelves of costumes, armour, and tons of theatrical paraphernalia. Out of curiosity I asked to see the cells and was politely shown them. There they were as of yore—the iron doors, with the little window or grating; but the doors were not locked, barred, and bolted—they were wide open, and the prison cells were occupied with sock and buskin.

Sir Thomas Henry was the main instrument in getting erected the spacious new Court opposite, in which he was never destined to sit. It was his ambition. Frequently had he said on the bench that the old court was a disgrace. I could not help thinking what Sir Thomas's opinion of the old Court would have been if he had seen it as I had just now. I could not help thinking the faithful old

Court had followed my example, and gone in for the stage.

Now it is razed to the ground, and there is not a brick left of the old place which, in my time, saw the preliminary examinations of the Flowery Land Pirates; Müller for the murder of Mr. Briggs; Barrett and others for blowing up Clerkenwell Prison; Burke and Casey; Dr. Hessell, who was acquitted on the charge known as the Great Coram Street murder, and on whose behalf Mr. Douglas Straight (now Mr. Justice Straight, of Allahabad) made the best speech he ever made in his life, I venture to think; the female impersonation case; and the charge against the police detectives Druscovich, Palmer, Meiklejohn, Clarke, and Mr. Froggatt, the solicitor, of assisting Kurr, Benson and others in committing the De Goncourt turf frauds. With the exception of the Pirates and Müller, *The Times'* reports were done chiefly by me.

The record of which I am most proud was in reference to a speech of Mr. Besley's in one of the above cases. He spoke for about seven hours, with one short interval, and as it proceeded I reported it in long hand, in the third person of course. To have done so *verbatim* would have been an impossibility. To have reported this speech with a pencil and paper would have been a tolerably easy matter, but I wrote it on manifold, producing twelve copies—that is, there were twelve oiled tissue sheets and six blank tissues between, altogether a thickness of eighteen papers to press through with the stylus.

To those uninitiated in the method of manifold writing, I can only explain that the system is the same as that adopted by cashiers in the stores and shops, who place a piece of black paper in a book, a little bill on the top, and by writing on the latter the impression is conveyed through the black to the book. Two copies are therefore procured. Imagine, therefore, the amount of pressure required for twelve copies, and the state of your fingers and hands after doing this with the utmost rapidity for seven hours with only about half an hour's cessation!

I may as well give a slight sketch of the characters of the three magistrates. Sir Thomas Henry was the very model of a police-court beak. He was tall and slim, and had natural dignity—a very different thing from the assumption of it. He was a good lawyer and a perfect courtier—not a mere police courtier. He liked approval, and whene'er he made a palpable hit in a passage of arms with an important counsel (specially retained), he would glance round the Court to see if it had been appreciated. After an effective summing up, the auditors in the body of the Court would sometimes break out with loud applause. Sir Thomas Henry would sternly observe that if such unseemly manifestations were again displayed, he should order the Court to be cleared. For all that, Sir Thomas liked that applause and was much gratified by it.

Mr. Frederick Flowers was a totally different type of man altogether. He was short, and had iron-grey hair and whiskers. He was exceedingly kind—much too kind for a magistrate, and possessed a dangerous talent for being humorous in Court. He hated to punish people and had a tendency to let everybody off—and did, if he could do so legally.

I remember once a woman, an old offender, being sentenced by one of the other magistrates to a month's imprisonment. On being removed from the dock by the gaoler she shouted, "Look here, the next time I am charged here I'll take jolly good care it's before old Flowers."

A little boy of about eight years of age was charged with snowballing an old gentleman. Mr. Flowers read the boy a kindly lecture, and told him never to snowball people in the streets again. As he had been detained in the gaoler's room for four hours and had been crying his eyes out, Mr. Flowers added that the child was evidently very sorry for what he had done, and would, therefore, be discharged. The mother who was advised to keep a better watch over her boy in future, came forward with profusions of thanks, and carried off the little prisoner in triumph. The prosecutor, who had watched the proceedings with amazement, here stepped into the box, and, addressing Mr. Flowers, said:

"Why, your worship, you've let him off."

*Mr. Flowers:* Of course I have.

*Prosecutor:* What for?

*Mr. Flowers:* You wouldn't have me punish a child like that, would you?

*Prosecutor:* Of course I would—what have I had him brought here for?

*Mr. Flowers:* I think he has been sufficiently punished.

*Prosecutor:* But look here—he has cut my cheek.

*Mr. Flowers:* Well, he did not do that on purpose.

*Prosecutor:* He snowballed me on purpose.

*Mr. Flowers:* Yes, but he didn't mean to cut your face.

*Prosecutor:* Well, he has done it, at all events.

*Mr. Flowers:* And he is very sorry, and so am I sorry; but I dare say when you were a boy you were in the habit of snowballing old gentlemen. At all events, I know I used to snowball people, and I am not going to fine any boy for doing what I used to do myself.

One morning a poor woman stepped into the box and expressed a wish to prosecute some man who had passed a bad sixpence upon her. Mr. Flowers took the counterfeit coin and after examining it said, "Well, I dare say the man didn't know it was a bad one: it is a remarkably good imitation of a genuine one. I'll tell you what I will do—I will give you a good sixpence in exchange; that will put an end to all legal proceedings." Mr. Flowers gave the woman a sixpenny-piece, and requested that the bad one should be broken up. When the Court was afterwards cleared, the good-natured magistrate, addressing me, said, "I hope, Mr. Grossmith, you won't think it necessary to report that case. If you do, I shall be having three or four hundred people coming to me to-morrow with bad sixpences to exchange."

A man was charged with violently assaulting his friend. A policeman saw the assault committed, and gave his evidence to that effect. The complainant, however, did not appear for the purpose of pressing the charge. When the constable had given his evidence, the defendant shouted out, "I didn't commit the assault. I never hit him."

*Mr. Flowers* (thinking this was the usual imputation on the evidence of the police): Then, if you didn't do it, who did I should like to know?

*Defendant:* I didn't do it. 'Twas the beer that did it.

*Mr. Flowers:* Oh, then we had better send the beer to prison.

*Constable:* Please, your worship, the complainant ain't here. He didn't wish to press the case.

*Mr. Flowers:* Oh, very well. *(To the Defendant)* There being no prosecutor, you and your friend the beer are discharged; but I should advise you not to become too closely associated with each other in the future.

In a series of articles which I contributed to *Punch*, at the beginning of the year 1884, entitled "Very Trying," I gave a skit of this magistrate. It was in the fourth article, and was headed "The Good-humoured Magistrate." He was extremely popular, and nobody, from his colleagues and counsel down to the prisoners themselves, was ever heard to say a harsh word against him.

Mr. James Vaughan (who still sits at Bow Street) was a solemn and severe type of magistrate. Absolutely just, and yet everyone seemed afraid of him. The just are always to be most feared. Mr. Vaughan makes a good magistrate, but he would have been a better judge. He has a power of "summing up" which is almost thrown away in a police court. He would give a decision (sometimes very elaborate) in every case that came before him. He was quite the reverse of a well-known magistrate of Great Marlborough Street, whose object was to get everything over as quickly as possible. I was once present at the last-named Court when there were a number of summonses against cabmen for delaying and obstruction. It was the custom to take all these summonses on one day. The mode of procedure adopted by this magistrate was as follows :

*Magistrate :* All those who plead guilty, step forward.

(Here about fifteen cabbies pushed to the front of the Court.)

*Magistrate :* Fined two shillings—don't do it again.

*(Exeunt* fifteen cabbies.)

Another magistrate, who used to sit at Worship Street, delivered his decisions in a species of shorthand. Suppose Smith and Brown were charged together with assaulting the police. At the conclusion of all the evidence the magistrate would say:

" Smith, five or five ; Brown, ten or fourteen ;" which, being interpreted, meant that Smith was to be fined five shillings, or in default of payment to be imprisoned for five days, and Brown to be fined ten shillings, or in default, fourteen days.

Now, Mr. Vaughan would certainly have read each man a serious warning, which (as Mr. Vaughan is a highly educated man) the prisoners may or may not have understood.

When I first went to the Court, I could not always understand his remarks, especially when some intricate technicalities were involved in them. In this predicament, I invariably went to his worship and asked if he would give me the principal points of his observations, a request on my part which was always met by Mr. Vaughan with much courtesy.

Mr. Vaughan was also a subject of my raillery in the *Punch* articles, from which I will give a short extract. A little boy of seven years of age is charged with begging, his excuse being he did not know he was doing any wrong. The magistrate delivers his decision in the following manner:

"Prisoner, you have been brought before me on the sworn testimony of a metropolitan constable, charged with begging within the precincts of the monument erected *in memoriam* to Nelson. It is, as you must be aware, a charge under the Vagrant Act, and I am bound to admit it appears to me there is a *prima facie* case against you. You have made no attempt to rebut the evidence of the officer, and I can only, as an *ultimatum*, give credence to his evidence, which admits of little doubt in my mind. The defence (if a defence it can be designated at all) that you have elected to set up is, to my mind, unworthy of the invention you have thought necessary to bestow upon it. You may not have perused the sections of the Act of Parliament bearing upon this particular charge, but every child must be aware, from maternal or paternal information, that the act of begging in any form is *contra leges*. Your defence is, therefore, totally unworthy of consideration. Now I warn you, if *in future* you will persist in pursuing this nefarious method of existence, I shall have to sentence you to a term of incarceration without the option of a pecuniary penalty. Pray do not treat this caution with indifference. Upon this occasion, however, your liberty will be afforded you.

"*The Prisoner* (in tears): Oh! how long have I got? Oh! what have I got?

"*Gaoler* (interpreting the learned magistrate): What have you got? Why, you've got let off, and don't do it again. *(Sotto voce* to the boy) Hook it!

"And the little boy left the Court, under the impression that the magistrate had sentenced him to several years' penal servitude, but that the gaoler had kindly overlooked the offence and liberated him."

Of course, this sketch is caricatured in the same way that the portraits in *Vanity Fair*, are by "Ape" (Mr. Carlo Pelligrini) and "Spy" (Mr. Leslie Ward).

Sir James Taylor Ingham succeeded to the post of chief magistrate at Bow Street on the death of Sir Thomas Henry, and was (and still is) a kind and considerate gentleman. It was the custom of some magistrates to wear their hats in Court, but I never saw this at Bow Street. At other Courts I have seen magistrates wear their hats; and one in particular I have seen walk about the bench with his hat on and his hands in his pockets, and never even remove it when a respectably-dressed woman was making an application to, or giving evidence before, him. If it were compulsory to keep the head covered, as when the judge assumes the black cap, one could understand it. But it is not compulsory, and there is no excuse for it, any more than there is for the young masher swaggering up a public dining-room where ladies are seated around dining, without having the common decency to remove his hat.

In 1877, when I appeared at the Opéra Comique, I retired from the work; but resumed it again in 1880, when my father died, having for my right-hand man Mr. Cleverley, whom my father had engaged to assist him. I retired eventually in favour of Mr. Cleverley, who is now *The Times* reporter; and if I possibly can help it, I will never give him a chance of "showing me up."

## CHAPTER IV.

### From Amateur to Professional.

---

"I once was a dab at Penny Readings."—*Ruddygore*.

---

"WHAT first put it into your head to give entertainments?" is a question I have been asked hundreds of times, and my reply has always been, "I'm sure I do not know." Nor do I know to this day. I used to play the piano very well at the age of twelve. What was considered "very well" for a boy twenty-eight years ago, no doubt would be considered execrable in these days of Hoffmanns and Hegners. I remember, when I played, ladies used to say, "How odd it seems to see a boy playing." It was thought effeminate to play the piano.

Besides playing from music, I also played a good deal by ear, which was considered demoralising, and still *is* by those who know nothing about it. Playing correctly by ear is a gift that should be encouraged. I was delighted one afternoon recently, when calling upon Mrs. Kendal, the well-known actress, to see her little boy, of about ten or eleven, sit down at the grand piano and play off by ear, perfectly correctly, "Le révenant de la revue" and one of my own songs. It is a gift delightful to the one fortunately endowed with it; and it does not follow that one should not also play correctly from music.

For my own pleasure (I do not know whether it was for other people's), I used to sing the comic songs, "Johnny Sands," "The Cork Leg," and "The Lost Child," to my own pianoforte accompaniment. I was never taught the tunes or words of these songs, but picked them up as children do, and reproduced them at the piano in a fashion of my own.

One delightful consequence of this was, that the number of my invitations to juvenile parties was considerably increased. I added to my stock of songs of course, and so found I was kept up to a late hour—at grown-up parties, too. Though not too young to learn and sing these songs, I was not old enough to always understand their purport.

There was a song, about this time, which was all the rage in London. The tune was heard on every organ and band, in every ballroom and theatre. I bought a penny song-book with the words, which I learned off by heart, and, as usual, picked out my accompaniment on the piano. One evening I launched it before the grown-up people who always turn up at the latter end of a juvenile party, and some of whom generally requested that I should be kept and made to sing to them. My friend Frank Burnand, in his incomparable *Happy Thoughts*, tells how he was singing a comic song before an unsympathetic audience, and suddenly remembering a verse was not quite proper, backed out of it. In my own case, I had no notion that the verse was *risqué*. I did not even understand it; so out it came with the full force of my penny-whistle voice. I never heard so much laughter in a room before. There was a general request for the song to be encored; but this was just a little too much for the feelings of my fond and hitherto proud mother, who made a dash at me, and shut me and the piano up at the same moment.

There is a period when the voice breaks, but I do not think I ever had a voice to break; at all events, I never remember the time when I ceased singing comic songs.

When half-way through my teens I began to write snatches of songs and illustrations, and received much help and encouragement from my father. He used to take me to the old Gallery of Illustration, to hear the inimitable John Parry; and this infused not only a new life, but a totally different style, into my work. Still in my teens, I used to be asked to the grown-up parties of Mr. Toole, Mr. Charles Millward, Mr. Henry Neville, and Mr. John Hollingshead, the last-named of whom, only the other day, reminded me that I never could be persuaded to sing before supper, excusing myself on the ground that the songs always went so much better *after* supper. So they did, and so they still do.

At Mr. Hollingshead's I first met Mr. Henry S. Leigh, then a contributor to *Fun*, and the author of "Carols of Cockayne," "Gillott and Goosequill," &c. He was himself a great admirer of John Parry; and when I became intimate with him, in after years, used to show me how Parry sang "Wanted, a Governess," "The Old Bachelor," "The Déjeuner à la Fourchette,"

&c., all of which I have myself sung at times, after a fashion. At Hollingshead's (in Colebrook Row), Leigh sang "The Twins," which became an enormously successful song, and he gave me a copy of it. Subsequently, I sang most of Leigh's songs *en amateur;* and after my appearance as a professional entertainer, he specially wrote "The Seven Ages of Song" and "The Parrot and the Cat" for me.

As a boy, I used, at certain evening parties, to accompany Toole in "A Norrible Tale" and "Bob Simmons," and considered it a high honour. I used to sing some of the songs of Henry J. Byron, a constant visitor to my father's house, and received much encouragement from him; also from John Oxenford, the dramatic critic of *The Times;* Andrew Halliday; T. W. Robertson, the dramatic author, and scores of others. It will be seen, therefore, that though I commenced on my own account, I was destined to be brought up in an atmosphere of literature and art. But neither my father nor myself was the first representative of the family on the public platform.

Judge Talfourd, the author of *Ion*, had heard my father recite over and over again, and strongly advised him to take up lecturing and reading as a profession. He followed the popular judge's advice, and gave his first lecture, entitled "Wit and Humour," on the day of my birth, at Reading, his native town. In a speech on the occasion of my coming of age he made use of these felicitous words: "I went down to Reading to make my first appearance in *public* at *my* native place, and, on my return, found my eldest son had made *his* first appearance in *private* at his native place."

That was forty years ago; but I propose presenting my readers with a copy of a programme, having reference to an uncle, dated twenty-five years before that. The programme is quaintly illustrated with tiny blocks of very primitive engravings, illustrating the characters personated:

BY PERMISSION OF THE WORSHIPFUL THE BAILIFFS.

NEW THEATRE, BRIDGNORTH.

For Two Evenings only.

On TUESDAY, the 26th, and Saturday, the 30th July, 1825.

Mr. GROSSMITH, sen., takes this opportunity of laying before the public the following high encomium passed on his son, kindly pointed out to him by a clergyman of Dudley. The numerous and repeated paragraphs which have appeared in all the London and provincial papers cannot have escaped the eye of anyone; but this work will, no doubt, escape the eye of some.

*Abstracted from the* "New Monthly Magazine," No. 45, July 1st, 1825 (page 299).

"The little Irish boy, Master Burke, betokens a dramatic instinct which can scarcely be mistaken. We saw in the country the other day a child, seven years old, named GROSSMITH, who displayed even a deeper vein of natural humour; actually revelling in the jests he uttered and acted; singing droll songs with the truth of a musician and the vivacity of a comedian; and speaking passages of tragedy with an earnestness and grace as though the dagger and bowl had been his playthings, and poetry his proper language."

Characters in the introduction which *Master Grossmith* imitates. (Here come in nine small illustrations of figures.)

Characters in *Pecks of Troubles* which Master Grossmith personates. (Here appear seven larger illustrations.)

THE CELEBRATED

INFANT

ROSCIUS,

MASTER GROSSMITH,

From Reading, Berks

(*Only seven years and a quarter old*),

Intends giving Two Evenings' Amusements, when he feels confident he will meet with that support he has never failed to experience in all the towns he has visited. The Infant Roscius will commence his performance with his

ADVENTURES IN THE READING COACH,

When he will imitate the following characters, namely: a Frenchman—a Fat Lady—an Affected Lady—a Tipsy Politician—a Stage Manager—Two Candidates for the Stage—and his own Success.

---

Master Grossmith will then go through the Humorous and Laughable Comedy of

PECKS OF TROUBLES;

OR,

The Distress of a French Barber.

---

(1) MISS DEBORAH GRUNDY
 (An Old Maid in Love) MASTER GROSSMITH!
(2) SPINDLESHANKS
 (A Dandy Fortune-Hunter) ... ... MASTER GROSSMITH!

(3) MONSIEUR FRIZEUR
   (In a Peck of Troubles
   about cutting old
   Grundy's face—
   with a song)   ... MASTER GROSSMITH!!!

(4) OLD GRUNDY
   (In search of the
   Frenchman, to give
   him a receipt in full
   for his carelessness) MASTER GROSSMITH!!!!

(5) BETTY, THE HOUSEMAID
   (In love with Corporal
   Rattle—with a song,
   "Yes, aye, for a
   Soldier's Wife I'll
   go")   ... ... ... MASTER GROSSMITH!!!!!

(6) CORPORAL RATTLE
   (As hot as gunpowder;
   in love with Betty) MASTER GROSSMITH!!!!!!

(7) TIMOTHY CLODHOPPER
   (A servant-of-all-work
   to old Grundy, be-
   wailing his unfor-
   tunate love for
   Betty, who has run
   off with Corporal
   Rattle — with the
   laughable song of
   "The Washing Tub,"
   which finishes the
   piece  ... ... ... MASTER GROSSMITH!!!!!!!

After which, "Betsy Baker," with other Comic Songs.

Part II. will consist of Scenes from the *Merchant of Venice, Douglas, Pizarro, Macbeth, Richard III., Rolla,* and *Hamlet.* The Infant Roscius will, on the first night, go through the tent scene of *Richard III.* The scenes will be changed each night, and he will conclude his performance with a piece (composed in two parts expressly for him) on

## THE MUSICAL GLASSES.

The whole of the scenery, wardrobe, and preparations, which are very extensive, with the Grand Diorama, 360 feet in length, will pass through the proscenium during the intervals of Master Grossmith's performance; consisting of views of Italy, &c.

---

Boxes, 3s.; Pit, 2s.; Gallery, 1s.

Doors to be opened at half-past Seven, and the performance to commence at Eight o'clock. Children under twelve and Schools, half price to Boxes and Pit only. Tickets and Plans for Boxes to be had of Mr. Gitton, Post Office; and at the Theatre, where Master G., and preparations, may be seen from Ten to One o'clock on the days of performance.

(Then appear four more blocks of the boy in private dress, and three Shaksperian characters.)

The above juvenile was Mr. William Grossmith, who, I am pleased to say, is still alive and well. He was the eldest of the male portion of the Grossmith family, and the only one remaining. He does not remember the entertainment with much pride or pleasure, and I do not wonder at it; for the work must have been a terrible strain upon the mind of a mere child.

I am in possession of several programmes similar to the above: and only the other day some kind stranger sent me a newspaper, dated Wednesday, June 17th, 1829, and called *The Bury and Norwich Post, or Suffolk and Norfolk Telegraph, Essex, Cambridge, and Ely Intelligencer.* One may well exclaim, "What's in a name?"

On glancing through its columns, I find the following :

## LINES
### ADDRESSED TO MASTER GROSSMITH.

Sure ne'er did Nature so profusely give,
Or such a Roscius till this time e'er live !
Deem it not flatt'ry, those who have *not* seen
This little wonder ! For full well, I ween,
Had you but view'd, like me, enchanted quite
You 'd own his genius, and in praise unite.
Ye who *have* seen the hero, ye can tell,
Tho' in his praise my numbers fain would swell,
Alas ! how feebly does my muse essay
His talents or his merits to portray.

Scarce ten years old ; superior strength of mind
Speaks in his "SPEAKING EYES" his sense refin'd :
His manners graceful, unassuming too ;
Such sweet simplicity we never knew :
So noble, free, and dignified his mien,
A real Hamlet seems to grace the scene.
When he with mimic art his skill applies,
And Shakspeare's heroes to assume he tries,
So well the child can personate the man,
That twenty years appear in one short span ;
Aye, not three minutes does the change require,
To make the maiden young or old, or 'squire.
But Shakspeare most his talents bring to sight :
There may experienc'd actors, with affright,
Think they ne'er more again must tread the stage,
While Grossmith is the Roscius of the age.
He weighs each word, and "*suits the action well ;*"
His rising its meaning oft will tell
Ere yet 'tis utter'd : his expressive face
Conveys the sense with ever-varying grace.
In short, no authors difficult appear
To his superior sense and gifted ear ;
His growing talents so conspicuous shine,
He gives a charm to Shakspeare's ev'ry line.

Farewell, sweet child ! May virtue guide thy way,
May bliss without alloy be thine each day,
And may'st thou e'er enjoy that peace of mind
Which dwells with virtue and with sense refin'd.

*Dowham Market, June 1st,* 1829.   M. M. C.

And now *revenons à nos moutons*.

At the close of 1864 I blossomed into a Penny Reader, and I can safely aver that no Penny Reader ever had such an exalted opinion of his own talents as I had of mine. Penny Readings were fast becoming the rage, and were springing up everywhere; and my first public appearance at them was in a schoolroom, in close proximity to Holy Trinity Church, Hawley Road, turning out of the Chalk Farm Road. This was the church I had been in the habit of attending, and in the choir of which I had sometimes sung. There was at Penny Readings no programme in those days. The chairman (always the vicar or the curate) used to call upon those in the audience whom he considered capable.

He flattered me with this distinction; so I took my seat at the piano, and sang a song with a refrain, in which the noisy portion of the audience commenced to join. This was not quite approved of; so for a time I contented myself with recitals from Dickens, Hood, &c., which I cribbed from my father's *repertoire*.

I soon returned to the comic songs again, but selected those of a milder form, like "He, She, and the Postman," a story without a chorus, and some out of Howard Paul's entertainment.

It was once suggested that we should give the short burlesque on *Hamlet* to which I have already referred. We arrived with several bags of costumes, which alarmed the vicar, and the performance did not take place. The audience, to our intense satisfaction, expressed its disappointment in an unmistakable manner;

so much so, that the chairman announced that it should be played on a future occasion. Meanwhile, he stipulated with me that there should be no costumes. I could not consent to this, and, after a long discussion, we met each other half-way. I was to be permitted to wear a cloak for Hamlet—or, rather, an old black shawl thrown over my shoulders. Horatio and the King were tabooed costumes. The Ghost (T. Bolton) was permitted to adorn himself with a clean tablecloth. My brother, who was only ten years of age, was to double the parts of Ophelia and Gravedigger. In the former, being so young, it was considered no harm for him to wear a muslin body and skirt; while, as the Gravedigger, he was allowed to take off his coat, and appear, for this occasion only, in his shirt-sleeves.

Somehow or other, Leclercq, the original representative of the Queen, could not appear, and I arranged with one of my schoolfellows from the North London Collegiate School to play the part. He had never acted before, and in all probability has never acted since. As he was about seventeen years of age, and looked a veritable young man, with a perceptible moustache, the vicar would not on any account allow him to assume ladies' attire. We eventually decided he should be allowed to throw a plaid shawl round his shoulders.

The eventful evening approached, and, as the intended performance had been whispered about, the rooms were crammed. All went well until the entrance of the Queen, late on in the piece which only played twenty minutes altogether. To the horror of the vicar, and to my own surprise, he had, behind the screen, slipped on a servant's cotton frock, and put on what is vulgarly known as a carotty wig. The vicar, who was, as usual, seated on the platform—a very small one, by-the-by,—rose and said in an undertone to me:

"I forbade this."

I replied that it was against my knowledge.

The performance went on, however; for the young man who played the Queen was such a stick that he was quite inoffensive, and uttered his words one after the other in the legitimate schoolboy fashion. But quiet people are always the most dangerous, and so it transpired with my young friend. We approached the finale, which, by the way, appears to me to be worth quoting. The characters are all lying on the stage, supposed to be dead.

HAMLET (*sitting up*)—
 What! Everybody dead? Why, that won't do;
 For who's to speak the tag? I must——

HORATIO (*rising*)— Not you.
 You've had your share of talking; so now stow it.
 I'll speak the tag——

KING (*jumping up*)— Not if I know it.
 *They've kept me back until the very last.
 Now, I'll speak the tag. Friends——

QUEEN (*getting up*)— Not so fast.
 Your notion, King defunct, is most absurd;
 The lady always utters the *last word!*

GHOST (*entering*)—
 Except when there's a goblin in the way.

OPHELIA (*entering*)—
 Then I, a female goblin, hold the sway.

HAMLET—
 Let's have a chorus, then—tune up—here goes:
 Sing to a tune that everybody knows

 * The King does not enter until the play scene, at the end.

Then followed a verse, to the catching air of "The Great Sensation." This we stood still and sung; but here it was that the representative of the Queen suddenly became overpowered with excitement, and could not restrain his feelings. What had hitherto been "reserved force" now became force without the slightest reserve. Irrespective of his costume, he danced violently and kicked wildly in the air. The audience indiscriminatingly laughed and applauded with delight! The vicar got up and held up his hands to the audience, to obtain silence, but without effect. He motioned to us to go off, and we all left the platform, with the exception of the Queen, who, positively mad with excitement, seized the reverend gentleman by the arms and swung him round two or three times. That was my last appearance at those particular Penny Readings.

I do not in the least despise Penny Readings. They are a very good school for beginners at all events.

At a party given at Manor Lodge, about 1869, John Oxenford, Andrew Halliday, and several others were all chatting to me about my songs, and advised me to get my father to write a short sketch, *à la* John Parry, to enable me to better introduce these sketches. The next year he did so. The sketch was entitled "Human Oddities," and lasted about forty minutes. I supplied the music: and the "Gay Photographer," since published, was one of the songs introduced; the words by G. G. *père*, and the music by G. G. *fils*. Dr. Croft, who then had great interest in the Polytechnic, and was, I fancy, one of the directors, introduced me to Professor Pepper, and I started on a trial trip on Nov. 11th, 1870; and observe, O ye superstitious ones, that I began on a Friday.

The following month I gave "The Yellow Dwarf," which I wrote myself, and which, I must admit, was exceedingly puerile. It was accompanied by dissolving views, and this Christmas entertainment was produced to oblige Prof. Pepper; but I did not relish being stuck at a piano in the corner and in complete darkness. If I am *not* seen, I am no good at all. I do not infer I am much good when I am seen. The only thing that went really well in "The Yellow Dwarf" was my setting of some words which appeared in *Punch*. The refrain, I remember, was:

<blockquote>
Faithful to Poll,<br>
Tol de rol lol ;<br>
Wherever he went he was faithful to Poll.
</blockquote>

It transpired that the words were written by F. C. Burnand, who has since become one of my most esteemed and valued friends, and who subsequently re-wrote them, and they were immortalised by Mrs. John Wood, under the title of "His Heart was True to Poll."

"The Yellow Dwarf" I continued for about a month, when, to my intense delight, "Human Oddities" was again put on, and ran about six months. In the autumn I produced "The Silver Wedding," and introduced the song - words by my father—"I am so Volatile."

Since then I have always written and composed my own sketches, which vary in length from about twenty to forty minutes, and, with very few exceptions, the words of the incidental songs. I do not sit down deliberately to write these. Ideas come to me in all sorts of places, and at most inconvenient times.

I wrote "He was a Careful Man" while travelling to Deal, and composed the music on the backs of envelopes on my return home. "The Muddle Puddle Porter" suggested itself to me while waiting for nearly an hour at Bishopstoke, and hearing an aged porter calling out the same string of stations. I wondered—supposing he obtained another "calling," such as a waiter who had to shout down a tube a string of dishes—whether he would not sometimes become confused by the recollection of his former situation, and mix up the names of the stations with the names of the joints. I am indebted very much to my old friend, Lionel Brough, for contributing so materially to the success of the song by his excellent singing of it.

I always write the words of the song first of course, and then the music. I composed over half a dozen tunes for "The Duke of Seven Dials" before I hit upon one to suit my fancy. I was a fortnight composing "The Lost Key," and only a couple of hours writing and composing "The Happy Fatherland." With regard to the "patter" portion of the sketch, that is the last part I write, and I alter it from time to time during its delivery—cutting out portions that do *not* "go," and extemporising observations and retaining them if they *do* "go."

Lots of people come to me and say, "I hope you won't take me off?" and I have replied that

I should never dream of doing such a personal thing : but I do, all the same ; and I have never known an instance where they have fitted the cap. If a very marked observation is made by a lady, I put it down to a gentleman, and *vice versâ*, though I often think the precaution quite unnecessary ; in proof of which I relate the following incident. As I was taking my seat at the piano, a lady, who evidently passed the entire season in attending about half a dozen afternoon parties daily, approached me and said : " I hope you are not going to be very long, Mr. Grossmith." This was said so innocently, and the remark so amused me, that I introduced it in the course of the sketch : the temptation was too great not to refer to it. The people roared with laughter, as they always do at anything personal to oneself. Personality always goes down better than pure wit. At the conclusion of the sketch I said to the lady:

" I hope I was not too long ? "

She replied, " Oh dear, no ; but did any lady really ask you that question ? "

I said, " Yes ; you did, if you remember."

" Did I ? " she replied.

"Most certainly."

" Yes," she continued, " but not with that comic expression."

" Of course not."

To return to the Polytechnic. I was regarded as the mild clown of the establishment, although I am bound to say that I thought some of the scientific and serious lectures far more humorous, unintentionally, than my work. On one occasion a lecturer was holding some explosive material in his hand, and said that its power was so great that, under certain conditions, it would blow up the whole of the Polytechnic Institution and the people in it. This announcement, delivered with much fervour, was rendered more alarming by the fact that the material was accidentally brought into contact with the spirit-lamp which stood on the table. The result was an insignificant "fizz," like a damp match.

During a discourse on the Franco-German war, the lecturer, explaining one of the views on the screen in which the French were defeated, gave vent to his own feelings in somewhat the following strain:

"Behold the cowards hewing down the poor French! That is not war—that is murder—miserable and uncalled-for murder!"

This strong sentiment called forth a hiss or two from some portions of the audience who happened to sympathise with the Germans. The lecturer held up his hands and said:

"Silence, my friends. Please remember that this is only a simple, unbiassed lecture, with pictorial illustrations of certain events which happened during this sad war. Do not let us show any personal feeling one way or the other."

There is little doubt that many of the lectures at the old Polytechnic were simply vehicles for introducing advertisements, just in the same way that, in the Pantomime Harlequinade, all the clown has to do is to bring on a box, which, on a touch from the wand of the harlequin, is turned into a magnified piece of popular soap, or a bottle of scent, with the name and address of the patentees printed in good-sized letters.

The following specimen is only a slight exaggeration of what I mean:

"Ladies and gentlemen, it is my pleasant duty this evening to give you a lecture on the beautiful city of Bombay; and, with the assistance of the magnificent dissolving views which I have at my command, the little trip which I propose to take in your company will prove almost as good as the reality to those who have *not* been fortunate enough to visit Bombay, and will recall most pleasant recollections to those who have. We will start by the ten o'clock express to Leeds. I am aware that this is somewhat out of the way, but it is worth while deviating a few hundreds of miles in order to travel by the new first-class carriages now running on the North South East Western line. This is, doubtless, the best line in the kingdom. I have no interest in the line whatever, although I quite appreciate the honour which the directors have conferred upon me by presenting me with a free pass. To return to the subject of Bombay. As one cannot leave this tight little island without crossing the dreadful Channel, I recommend those of my audience who are not good sailors to procure a tin of 'Bankem's Anti-Seasick Biscuits;' they are an infallible remedy, and can be procured at Brown's in Cheapside, Jones's at Charing Cross, and Robinson's in Piccadilly. My sole reason in mentioning this, is the comfort of the British public. Well, eventually we reach Bombay, and there is a deal to see. You should get one of 'Jidson's double binocular, concave, magnifying, four-jointed field glasses.' The next four views are of 'Messrs. Jidson's

Warehouses in the City.' The pavements being hot in Bombay, I should recommend your taking a pair of 'Shoeling's leather-sandalled, woollen-lined bluchers.' There is no boot manufacturer's to equal these bluchers for walking abroad. If you enquire at the door, at the conclusion of the lecture, they will give you Messrs. Shoeling's card and circular of full particulars. I have often wondered why, in an enterprising city like Bombay, they have never laid down ' Johnson's Tar Macadamised Wood Pavements.' The next view is an instantaneous photograph of Messrs. Johnson's *employés* laying down the pavement in Scent Street, Bermondsey. This pavement is more successful than any other ever tried in the vast metropolis. Their agent is James Wilkins, 19A Stone Buildings. On arriving at Bombay, I should suggest your going to the 'Golden Hawk,' English hotel; proprietor, Mr. Mulgan Jackson, a most civil landlord. The prices are moderate; and you can have an early bath, if you wish, although I should advise your taking with you a 'Scalden's folding indiarubber douche bath.' They take up little room, and only weigh a couple of hundredweight. Do not take candles with you, for they melt in Bombay immediately. Take a 'Flamer's duplex paraffin fusel lamp,' a sample of which I produce for your inspection. As you may not be able to get the right oil in Bombay, you will be compelled to take a few gallons with you; and, while I think of it, if you want to write home, get from Mr. Williams, 290 Bridge Street, Marylebone Square, a ninepenny 'Multum in Parvo,' which contains a writing tablet, bottle of 'undryupable ink,' a quire of note-paper (four different tints), envelopes to match, four steel pens, two quill ditto and wiper, wafers, ink-eraser, stick of sealing-wax, and an almanack. Ladies and gentlemen, the next view, a photograph of 'Wheeler's double-tyred tricycle,' will conclude the first of my series of six lectures on Bombay. I thank you for your kind attention. The diving-bell will now descend in the great hall, and, on your way there, please don't forget to look at the stall containing specimens of 'Messrs. Glasse's folding perambulators,' as they may be useful if you desire to take your children with you to Bombay."

Alas! the lecturer in town and country seems to have had his day. When I was a boy, there were hundreds of lecturers on thousands of subjects. During the winter months there were lecturers everywhere. Elderly people went to be instructed; young men and women to "eye" each other; while boys went invariably to be "turned out."
Dissolving views were the most patronised of the serious lectures, and I do not think I ever went to one at which some unfortunate person was not ejected. The darkness tempts unruly people to interrupt. It is with much pain and regret that I confess to having been myself politely requested to leave the Polytechnic (before I was engaged there) for unseemly conduct. On one occasion the lecturer was stating, amidst breathless silence, "This particular bark is infested with ten thousand millions of parasites." I simply said, in a high

falsetto, "Oh, indeed!" The lights were turned up, and I was turned out!

Professor Pepper always took most kindly to me, and it was his only disappointment, I believe, that I could not introduce the immortal ghost-effect in my humorous *scénas*.

In the spring of 1871 I produced "The Puddleton Penny Readings," and in the autumn "Theatricals at Thespis Lodge." That was my last engagement there; for Dr. Croft came into power, and wrote most of the humorous entertainments himself. These were designed entirely for the magic lantern, and had, therefore, to be given in the dark. I naturally could not see my way to undertake them, and reluctantly refused his kind offer to stay on.

One little story, and I bid farewell to the old Polytechnic.

Professor Pepper was a perfect adept at satisfying an audience; if by chance the experiments went wrong; and sometimes they *did* go wrong, and no mistake, in the good old days, at the Polytechnic. I shall never forget the first-night failure of an entertainment called "The Arabian Mystery," and the manner in which Professor Pepper, by good temper and chaff, prevented a crowded audience from being very disagreeable. "The Arabian Mystery" may be explained as follows: One girl was blindfolded and placed on the platform, with her back to the audience. A large screen was then placed so as to conceal her from the public. Another girl walked down the centre aisle with a pack of cards, and then waited the Professor's orders. Professor

Pepper then produced a white board, about four feet long by two and a half wide, on which appeared in black some hieroglyphics that I have no hesitation whatever in denouncing as sham. After dwelling on the mysteries of this supposed Arabian fable, or whatever it was, Professor Pepper threw it on to the stage in front of the screen. (I may mention that the entertainment took place in the small theatre which some years afterwards was burned down.) The audience tittered considerably when the board of hieroglyphics was pitched upon the stage; and Pepper, with great solemnity, called to the poor girl, who was standing amongst the audience in a great state of nervousness, and instructed her to request some lady or gentleman to "select a card." Someone chose a card, and handed it back to the girl, who walked at once to a particular spot in the aisle, and, by means of a series of pressures of the foot (which were perceptible to everyone in front of the house), tried to convey the name of the card by electricity to the girl behind the screen. There was a long pause, and no reply; during which Professor Pepper said to the girl in front:

"No wonder she does not tell you the name of the card, for you have not asked her to do so."

There were a few ironical cheers then, which only succeeded in making the poor girl more nervous than ever.

Professor Pepper again addressed her, saying:

"You had better give her another card, and let us try again. The audience must remember that this is the first night of 'The Arabian Mystery,' and some little allowance should be made."

This observation brought forth the usual applause; which shows that a British audience is always game for fair play.

Another card was offered, taken, and returned to the girl, who, as before, walked back to the same spot, and once more tried with her foot to convey the message to the platform, at the same time asking, in a tremulous voice, "What card do I hold up?"

The card happened to be the ace of diamonds. After a pause, the girl behind the screen, in a shrill voice, shouted, "Seven of clubs!"

The audience, being perfectly good-tempered, simply roared with laughter at the fiasco.

Professor Pepper placed his hands up, to suggest that they should be silent, but for a considerable period he was unsuccessful in procuring order. When he could be heard, he said:

"Ladies and gentlemen, I dare say you are of opinion that the lady behind the screen has made a mistake." (Loud laughter.) "As it happens, she is perfectly correct! This is an Arabian mystery, and I ought to have explained to you that in Arabia the ace of diamonds *is* the seven of clubs."

This preposterous joke was greeted with applause and laughter.

Professor Pepper (continuing) said: "That is right. I am glad to see that such good feeling exists between us. Now, we'll try again, please. Offer another card."

Whether the next few attempts were successful I cannot remember. I was not so interested, I am sorry to say, in the successful attempts as in the failures. But I am quite certain with regard to the result of the last card offered. It was (we will say) the three of clubs. The girl behind the screen shouted, "Queen of hearts." This was a little too much; and though half the audience still took this failure in good part, the other half showed unmistakable signs of impatience.

Professor Pepper, with perfect good humour, said:

"Ladies and gentlemen, I must ask for your consideration again. You seem to forget that this is an Arabian mystery. Now, if the lady behind the screen told you correctly the name of the card, there would be no mystery about the matter, for the trick is a very simple one. Anybody can do it. But the 'mystery' is, how is it she is *not* telling the cards correctly? *That's* the Arabian mystery, and no mistake."

Owing to the cheery manner of the popular lecturer, and a promise that it should be "all right" the next night, the audience departed to the large theatre, to hear Mr. George Buckland, who was a great favourite at the Polytechnic Institution.

## CHAPTER V.

### In the Provinces.

"A wandering minstrel I."—*The Mikado.*

I CONCLUDED my first long engagement at the Polytechnic in the summer of 1871, and Mr. and Mrs. Howard Paul engaged me to join them for several weeks on a seaside tour. This was to me a delightful way of combining business with pleasure, and I particularly remember a delightful week at Scarborough.

I returned to the Polytechnic in the autumn, and produced "The Silver Wedding," a short easy version of which I have published. It was in this sketch I introduced "I am so Volatile," which was the first comic song I published. Applications were continually made to me from provincial institutions; but I could only accept those at a short distance from town, as my daily work at Bow Street had to be done as well. It was hard work; but I am used to hard work, and enjoy it.

All prospects of entering for the Bar disappeared, and it was my father's own suggestion that we should try an entertainment together. He was an enormous favourite in the country as a humorous reciter; and he thought my piano and songs would prove more attractive if given with him, as it might otherwise have been thought that I was starting a rival entertainment — a thought which neither of us desired to encourage.

We accordingly worked out a trial programme, and in May, 1873, we gave our joint recitals at the Masonic Hall, Birmingham. The papers of May 12th spoke most highly of the entertainment; and the result was, my father decided that in the autumn we should start together with a tour of the provincial institutions. As I previously stated, I had only visited institutions which I could conveniently reach after my daily work at Bow Street; but as I was married on May 14th, two days after the above trial trip, it became necessary for me to materially increase my income.

I was fortunate in having the permanent assistance at Bow Street of Mr. H. R. Hollingshead, son of Mr. John Hollingshead, the popular manager and author; so there was no longer a bar to a continued tour. First of all, there was my honeymoon to be spent. To take a trip abroad was quite beyond my means, and no noble Duke in those days came forward to place his country demesne at our disposal; so, amidst a shower of rice, my wife and I departed for Leamington. Why Leamington? Well, I will tell you. I had received a very good offer from my friend, Mr. Wm. Southern, of that town, who thought it would be a good thing for me to give a single-handed recital at the end of the fortnight I intended staying, and he would see that the interesting circumstance of my passing my honeymoon was carefully paragraphed in the papers. The result was a crowded room, and the cost of my pleasure trip materially reduced.

We visited other places, and wound up our happy month at the charming residence of one of my wife's relatives at Aigburth, near Liverpool. Here was another stroke of business on my part; for I joined forces with Mrs. Howard Paul in a combined entertainment for a week, at the Concert Hall, Bold Street, Liverpool. In the autumn, however, the tour with my father commenced. We started in Devonshire and Cornwall, the result being that I was away from home a fortnight. We usually got home on Saturdays, that being no day for the institutions. I did not at all like leaving the girl I loved behind me, and I always disliked (and suppose I always shall) travelling.

I append a programme of one of the recitals given in conjunction with my father during the season 1872-3:

BIRKBECK LITERARY AND SCIENTIFIC
INSTITUTION,

Southampton Buildings, Chancery Lane.

---

PROGRAMME
OF THE
LITERARY AND MUSICAL ENTERTAINMENT
TO BE GIVEN BY
MESSRS. GEORGE GROSSMITH,
ON WEDNESDAY EVENING, JUNE 9TH,
Commencing at Half-past Eight o'clock.

---

PART I.
Mr. GEORGE GROSSMITH.
GEMS FROM CHARLES DICKENS
(In Memoriam).
Little Tony Weller and his Grandfather.
Birth of the Junior Partner in the firm of "Dombey and Son"

### PART II.
**Mr. GEORGE GROSSMITH, Jun.**
A New Descriptive Melody, entitled—
## "SEVEN AGES OF SONG!"
And (by request) Selections from his Humorous and Mimetical Sketch, entitled—
## "THE PUDDLETON PENNY READINGS."

### PART III.
**Mr. GEORGE GROSSMITH.**
## THE HUMOUR OF MARK TWAIN.
Autobiographical Reminiscences.
Our first Visitor.
Journalism down in Tennessee.
&c., &c.

### PART IV.
**Mr. GEORGE GROSSMITH, Jun.**
New Musical Scena,
## "IN THE STALLS!"
Annual Invitation—Up to London—Lord Mayor's Show in a Fog—Stalls at the Pantomime—Science at the Polytechnic—High-class Music (never performed out of London)—"Our daily work is over."

Admission, 6d.   Pit, 1s.   Reserved Seats, 2s.   Members free.

I also attach one of my single-handed programmes:

### ALEXANDRA CLUB AND INSTITUTE,
Truro Road, Wood Green.

R. D. M. LITTLER, Esq., Q.C., President.

### ENTERTAINMENTS FOR MEMBERS & FRIENDS.

The next of the above Entertainments will take place on
WEDNESDAY, DECEMBER 31, 1873.
LITERARY AND MUSICAL ENTERTAINMENT
BY
## Mr. GEO. GROSSMITH, Jun
(Of the Royal Polytechnic, London Concerts, &c.)

## PROGRAMME.

Original Colloquial and Pianoforte Sketch, entitled—

### "OUR CHORAL SOCIETY."

Musical Movement in Moreton-super-Mire—Great Excitement, Local and Vocal—Moreton acquires a Choir—Formation of the Society—The pleasure of Singing (and the pain of Listening)—The Patroness, Lady Alum Gargle—Her Harmonic Triumphs, past and present—The Society gets up a Public Bawl for the benefit of a Private Charity—A Polite Conductor—Mr. G. Sharp composes a new Cantata, "The Penitent Pilgrim"—The Pilgrim undergoes a trying Rehearsal—The Concert!—Marvellous effect of an indistinct "Reapers' Chorus"—Breathless effect of the long runs—The Secular Music—Pianoforte Solo by Miss Spikes—Manufacture of Italian Songs—Grand Finale, "Lightly Tripping o'er the Hills," by Mr. and Mrs. Hoggsedd.

### READINGS.

THE "CORONER'S INQUEST," by THOMAS HOOD,

And an original, humorous narrative (after ARTHUR SKETCHLEY), entitled

"MRS. BROWN on the SHAKSPERIAN DRAMA."

OLD SONG ... ... "My Dejeûner à la Fourchette"... ... JOHN PARRY

To conclude with a New Musical and Whimsical Fancy, entitled,

### "JOTTINGS FROM THE JETTY."

To commence at Eight o'clock precisely.

Tickets (Non-members), 6d. Reserved Seats, 1s. 6d.
May be obtained at the POST OFFICE, Wood Green; BARKER'S LIBRARY, Commercial Road; and at the CLUB ROOM, Truro Road.

### MEMBERS FREE,

Who may also obtain one Lady's Ticket for Sixpence on application to the Manager at the Club only.

F. WOOD,
G. DEMANT, } Hon. Secs.

These years of tearing about all over the United Kingdom were more or less amusing—"generally *less*," as H. J. Byron observed. The visits with my father were the most varied. With Mrs. Howard Paul or Miss Marryat, costumes were introduced, and the entertainment appealed to a broader section of the public. When with my father, the entertainment was patronised by the more serious section of the public. He would be giving recitals from *Pick-*

*wick* and *David Copperfield*, with my comic songs and sketches alternating, on a small platform with four or five clergymen seated thereon, they being perhaps the Committee. I always got on very well with the clergy; in fact, I have always regarded myself as a species of religious comic singer. After the recitals the Committee would follow us into the ante-room; four would engage my attention, while the fifth —generally a young curate—would surreptitiously slip the fee into my father's hand. I remember him once upsetting the solemnity of this "settling-up" proceeding by exclaiming loudly, "I am not ashamed of being paid. You need not hand me the fee as if it were an election bribe."

My father had frequently suggested that the moment I arrived in a town I should look through the local papers, for the purpose of introducing some special topics that would come home to that particular place in the course of my sketches, which easily admitted of *ad libitum* observations. I always intended doing it, knowing how well local topics are received; but, somehow or other, I kept forgetting to carry out my intention.

One night, however, a splendid opportunity presented itself. It was some place in the Midland Counties, and an Alderman, whom we will call Juggins, had got into terrible hot water through proposing to have removed from the middle of the main thoroughfare an old stone pump. The local papers devoted columns to the controversy. Half the townspeople held that the pump was sacred to them—it was a monument, an ancient landmark, it was everything useful and ornamental. The other half disagreed. The only opinion in which the townspeople were unanimous was that, whether right or wrong, Alderman Juggins had nothing to do with it, and that he was simply advertising himself.

The evening arrived, and the hall was full. My father occupied the first half-hour, commencing at eight, with a selection from *Adam Bede.* I arrived at half-past eight, and in five minutes stepped on the platform, and commenced with my old sketch, " The Silver Wedding." The sketch concludes with a description of the supper, and the toasts proposed in honour of Mr. and Mrs. Alphonzo de Brown's silver wedding, &c., &c., with the responses. In the imitation of an old friend of the family, I spoke as nearly as I can recollect, as follows: " We all congratulate our dear host and hostess on having arrived at this important epoch in their lives, and the occasion has created even more sensation than that created by Alderman Juggins's pump." I waited for the tremendous roar of laughter and applause that would surely follow this remark. To my intense surprise, there was not the ghost of a laugh. It could only be accounted for in one way—I had evidently dropped my voice, and the " gag " had consequently missed its mark. I would try again.

I proceeded with the supposed old gentleman's speech, and concluded thus : " We will drink the toast upstanding all, with three times three ; we will drink it in bumpers—we will drink it with wine, good wine, such as only our host can give—

wine that has not been diluted by the product of Alderman Juggins's pump." This time I shouted the last sentence, so that there should be no mistake about their hearing it. To my horror, not a smile. Something was wrong! Perhaps the observation was out of place in the old gentleman's speech.

I would not be beaten; so I determined to give it another chance in the comic man's speech. I rattled off the following nonsense in the character of the humorous gentleman: "Well, in returning thanks for the ladies, I may say I am very fond of them"—(laughter)—"and I think I may also say that they are very fond of me." (Roars of laughter.) "My only regret is, that I am not in a position to marry all the dear ladies who are round this festive board to-night." (Continued hearty laughter, an elderly lady and a curate in the front now nearly going into hysterics. Some people, fortunately, are easily pleased.) "Bless the ladies! If I thought I had ever done a single act to incur their displeasure, I would immediately go out of the house and drown myself in Alderman Juggins's pump!"

The effect was electrical. The enthusiastic audience immediately became depressed, and someone at the back of the hall shouted, "Ha' done with that pump, lad—we've had enough of it!"

My heart sank into my boots, and I could scarcely sing the song, "I am so Volatile," which usually concluded the sketch. I retired to the ante-room, and instantly attacked my father. I said, "Well, I have taken your advice, and introduced a topic, with the result that it was a dead failure. I shall take good care never to repeat the experiment."

My father said, "Topic? What topic?"

"Why," I responded, "I made several allusions to the Juggins's pump discussion, with the result that I made a complete ass of myself."

My father burst out laughing, and said, "I don't wonder at it. Didn't you hear me do it? Why, I worked it up all through the first part."

"But," I argued, "how could you do that? You were reciting *Adam Bede*."

"I know I was," he answered. "I kept bringing Alderman Juggins's pump in Mrs. Poyser's remarks, and it went *enormously*."

I do not know what the feelings of the audience were, but I leave the reader to imagine mine.

Country audiences are certainly most enthusiastic and delightful to entertain. Of course there are exceptions, and the following is an amusing one:

We were at some little hall in the country, and when my father concluded the first portion of the entertainment he said to the chairman, who followed him into the ante-room:

"The audience seem most enthusiastic."

The Chairman replied: "Do you think so, Mr. Grossmith? Why, I thought they were exceptionally apathetic."

My father replied: "Well, I thought they were, if anything, *too* enthusiastic; for they were knocking their umbrellas and sticks, without cessation, on the ground all the time."

The Chairman replied, languidly: "Oh, that wasn't applause. You see, our post-office is at the other end of the room, and they are simply stamping the letters for the up mail."

The usual fee at the institutions was five guineas. There were a few that could afford more; but against this there was a good fifty per cent. of institutions that begged of the lecturers to knock off a guinea or two. Some were not quite so exacting, and begged that only the "shillings" might be deducted.

My father used to relate an amusing adventure he had experienced concerning the reduction of fees. At some out-of-the-way spot in Scotland he was met on the railway platform by a deputation of old gentlemen, who conducted him to his hotel. At twenty minutes to eight o'clock this Scotch deputation came to the hotel and conducted him to the lecture-hall. After the lecture, the same elderly deputation conducted him back to the hotel. The next morning, having ascertained the hour at which he meditated departing, the deputation turned up again, and conducted him back to the station. On the platform the elder man of the deputation, addressing my father, said:

"You'll be sorry to hear that we find, on making up the accounts, we are exactly £1 14s. 6d. out of pocket by your lecture. We thought you would not like to leave the town with that upon your mind; and so we give you the opportunity of returning the deficit, and enabling you, with a clear conscience, to say we have not lost by your visit."

My father, in telling this story, used to add:

"I told the deputation it was most kind of them to afford me the opportunity, and I certainly would carefully consider the matter. I kept my word; for, although that occurred ten years ago, I have been carefully considering it ever since."

When my father and I appeared together, a double fee was demanded; but this was sometimes alleviated on the "reduction-on-taking-a-quantity" principle. Some institutions could not engage us; and assuming always that these could stand the entertainment, but not the fee, we used to part for a night or two and go our divers ways, and join forces again at the next town where both were engaged. The lecture season used to last about seven months. We had to pay our own railway fares and hotel bills, of course; but as we travelled third, and lived very moderately, the expenses were not great.

Then my father, being so popular socially, was nearly always entertained, and, for his sake, the hospitality was frequently extended to me; and I take this opportunity to express my gratitude to the many strangers in the country who have offered me a home, made me very comfortable, and saved me an hotel bill. After the lectures we often were taken home to supper, and some of the audience or friends of the host asked to meet us, and my father used to keep the whole table in a roar. It was, of course, on account of his popularity that on arriving in a town there was a little rush to secure us as guests. Sometimes there was a rush in the opposite direction; but hospitality generally held the sway. The Secretaries used to write:

"Dear Sir,—Mr. Blank, our Mayor, desires the honour of entertaining you. Personally I am sorry, for I had hoped to have entertained you myself.
"Yours, &c., &c."

Precedence was always given to the Mayor, and very jolly fellows the provincial Mayors are. In one town I was always "roofed" by the Mayor—the same Mayor. As far as I can say, he always had been elected Mayor, and always would be. It appears that there sometimes is a great difficulty in persuading anybody to be the Mayor. Certainly there is no eagerness displayed in some towns to secure that official position. The Librarian of a town, who was selling tickets for my entertainment, said:
"Our Mayor, Mr. Z——, who entertains you here, Mr. Grossmith, has made himself so popular by his liberality that we shall elect him again next year. The last Mayor never spent a single penny of the allowance made him."
"How much does a Mayor get here?" I asked.
"Ten pounds," said the Librarian, "and Mr. Z—— has spent nearly the whole of it on banquets, &c."

I have frequently been asked, in reference to the long runs at the Savoy Theatre, if I have not derived some interest from the change of audiences. It appears to me that the audiences at the Savoy are always the same, except in numbers. The house may not be so full, and the enthusiasm may vary; but in all other respects they are the same. When I give my entertainments at the Savoy, the same points tell, and the laughter and applause come in exactly the same places. In the country I never quite knew what would take. I am speaking of the general patter.

Things that missed fire in London went enormously in the country; but I am bound to say that, taken altogether, I have been much flattered by the gracious way in which my sketches have been received in all places and by all kinds of people. I have experienced extraordinary changes in the style of audience. I gave the same selection in the drawing-room of the Duchess of St. Albans, before T. R. H. the Prince and Princess of Wales and about two dozen other distinguished ladies and gentlemen, in March, 1874, that I gave, a few days after, at Falkirk, to about 1,500 enthusiastic Scotch people, the greater part of whom had paid the admission charge of one penny. The selection included my sketches of Amateur Theatricals, a Christmas Pantomime, the Penny Readings, &c.

I have not often been interrupted in public rooms. In private, I have by people talking. But whenever I am interrupted, I make a point of remonstrating. I do not adopt this course for the mere sake of what is vulgarly called "side," or "swagger," but because my nerve absolutely fails me if I become distracted. The moment I become nervous, I am, so to speak, wrecked.

I feel a little diffident in telling the following story, inasmuch as it shows myself to advantage. I was giving an entertainment at Greenwich with Mrs. Howard Paul. I was singing a song called "Awfully Lively," in character, accompanied by Miss Blanche Navarre, the singer, who remembers the incident well, when I was much put out by a "funny man" in the back seats, which were very high up, I being on a platform low down, as if in a well. He commenced with a comic laugh in the wrong place. The audience tittered audibly. A little later on he interrupted with a comic cough. The audience laughed outright, and so they did again with increased vigour when he subsequently indulged in a comic sneeze. I determined to take no notice of it, thinking he would get tired. Not a bit of it. He next treated me to a comic remark which completely put me off, and I broke down in the middle of my song. Quietly addressing the audience, I said: "Ladies and Gentlemen,—There are two comic gentlemen here to-night, and you cannot very well hear both at the same time. It would be extremely selfish on my part were I to entirely monopolise the platform to the exclusion of the other comic gentleman; therefore, with your kind permission, I will retire for a short time, and give him the opportunity of coming down here and giving his entertainment. When he has finished, I will resume."

I then retired from the platform, but listened at the door to hear what was going on. I heard cries of "Go down!", "Sing a song!" amid laughter and applause. But being funny in an audience and being funny on a platform are two distinct things; and the difference was evidently appreciated by the other comic gentleman, who absolutely declined to accept the invitation to "go down" or to "sing a song." I then heard my own name called repeatedly, so I returned to the platform and met with a good reception. When silence reigned, and as I perceived good humour prevailed, I said: "The other comic gentleman having exhausted his stock of humour, I will proceed with mine." This was received with cheers, and subsequently all was peace.

I was obliged to resign a proposed prolonged engagement with Mrs. Howard Paul; for her tours would take her away from London months at a time, while the entertainment with my father always brought me home on Saturday night, and sometimes would allow of my being weeks in London at a time: so from 1873 till 1876 I visited the institutions with him when possible, and by myself when not.

Sometimes I used to make my single-handed engagements fit in capitally—sometimes I did not. To fill up five consecutive days in Yorkshire, including the institutions at Leeds and Bradford, who always paid the full fee, with a request that I should visit them again the following season, was most satisfactory.

But such a happy state of things could not always be arranged. The usual course was this: The first good offers that came in were "booked" immediately, no matter what part of the United Kingdom they came from. The next applications had to be fitted in. Sometimes I managed to fit in, say, Monday, Wednesday, and Thursday in

Cornwall and Devonshire. Tuesday would be vacant, and rather than lose the day I would arrange, at a reduced fee, to give an entertainment at some very small institution. As a matter of advertisement that is a very bad thing to do. The larger institutions hear of it, and naturally expect you to do the same for them.

Occasionally, through mismanagement or ill-luck, the engagements were arranged in a dreadfully inconvenient manner. Twice in one season I had to entertain in Edinburgh one night and London the next.

One of these nights I shall not easily forget. I was singing at the private residence of a then popular Bailie, in Edinburgh. I hurried from the house to catch the night mail to London. The snow was terrible, and I got into a third-class carriage, tipping the guard to try and keep the compartment for myself, as I wanted to change my evening clothes for a warmer suit. The guard said, "All right, sir," took the tip, locked the door, then immediately unlocked it again and ushered in a drunken ruffian of the lowest type. There were no cushions to the seats of the third class carriages in those days, so I took out my two air-cushions—one to sit upon and the other to put at the back of my head. I began to blow them out, and as they expanded, the ridiculous operation evidently tickled the fancy of my distinguished fellow-passenger, who began to grin and chuckle in an idiotic fashion. Thinking that after all he was a good-tempered fellow, I asked him if he had any objection to my changing my things.

He leered at me and asked, "What for?"

I said I had on a thin evening suit, that it was a bitterly cold night, and that I wanted to attire myself in something warmer.

"You shan't do it if I can help it!" he said sulkily, and at the same time he shifted along the seat till he was exactly opposite to me. As there was no chance of the train stopping till we got to Carlisle, my feelings may be imagined. "Change your clothes, indeed," he kept muttering; "not while I'm here."

I felt much vexed, and yet saw he was a very ugly customer to cross in temper. He began to fill his pipe, and I seized the opportunity to observe:

"I don't object to your smoking, although this is not a smoking carriage."

He replied, "I'm not going to ask you whether you object or not."

"Very well, have your own way," I remarked.

"I mean to," he grunted, and for the next quarter of an hour puffed away in silence. He was evidently thinking. So was I. I was thinking that if I had been the same size and weight as my delightful companion, we might have come to better terms. Presently he said, "What do you want to change your clothes for?"

"I told you," I replied, "I feel cold, and want to put on something warm."

"Well, I'm not going to let you," he said.

"I know! You said that before," I remarked.

"And I'll say it again. Do you hear?" he shouted. "I'll say it again. I'm not going to let you. There! How do I know who you are? It's only thieves and murderers who go about changing their clothes.  I don't say you are one : still, how am I to know you are *not* one—eh ?  Tell me that."

I ventured no observation whatever, but let him go on.  He evidently was working himself up into a species of fever, and feeling oppressed let down the window, and in came a hurricane of wind and snow.  Now when a man of this description is drunk and inclined to be violent, there is only one method of procuring temporary peace.  No matter how drunk he is, hand him a brandy-flask.  I therefore took down my bag and opened it.  Whether the man thought I was looking for a revolver or not I cannot say, but he watched my proceedings with suspicion and carefully drew from his pocket a large clasp-knife, which he opened and placed on the seat beside him.  This opened my eyes considerably to the kind of customer I had to deal with.  I found the flask, and poured into the metal cup about a large wine-glassful of neat brandy.

Addressing him, I said : " You're a disagreeable fellow.  You want to quarrel with me, but I tell you plainly I am not going to quarrel with you.  So drink this."

The beast (one could scarcely call him a man) took the cup and drained the brandy.  In the meanwhile I pulled up the window, a proceeding to which my friend said he had not the "slightest objection."  Suddenly there was a loud *whirrrr*, and I was jerked forward on my seat by the sudden application of the brake to the train.  We slackened pace and eventually pulled up at some little dark station, the signal evidently being against us.  Before I could get to the door on the left side, the man had crossed and let down the window.

I shouted to the fellow, "Here! get out quickly; I'll stand you another drink."

He got out on to the platform and staggered off the length of the carriage, presuming I was following. The guard rushed up and called to the man to get back, as "the train was not stopping at that station." This was scarcely the truth, but I knew what he meant.

I stood on the step and stopped the guard, saying: "You ought to be ashamed of yourself, after taking a 'tip' from me, to put a drunken brute like that into the carriage."

The man on the platform began shouting after me, "Come on, mate!"

The guard locked my door and proceeded to get the man into another carriage. The man would not go.

I heard the guard say, "If you don't get in here, you'll be left behind."

The man pushed the guard away and made for my carriage again. The guard followed and a short tussle ensued, the man striving to open the locked door of my carriage, with a few choice expressions that eclipsed even the worst that I had been accustomed to hear in Bow Street Police Court. The end of it all was, that the guard lost his temper and the man lost the train.

Another unfortunate arrangement of dates was, London one night, Monmouth the next night, and somewhere in the North the third, involving my return to London first before proceeding there. The journey to Monmouth was the coldest I ever recollect. I did not arrive until close upon eight o'clock. The entertainment was given in conjunction with my father, who happened to be lecturing in that district. He instructed me, on arrival, to go to the hotel. When I got there I was instantly served with a chop, fresh from the grill, and a small bottle of Guinness. My father, ever thoughtful for my comfort, had arranged for my favourite meal, and left a little note, in shorthand, for me to this effect: "My dear old boy, take your time. I will go on till I see you are in the hall.—Your ever affectionate Guv."

He had to open the proceedings, as usual when we gave the joint recitals, and he meant by the above note that he would go on reciting until he knew I was prepared to give one of my musical sketches. I finished my simple dinner and walked over to the hall. By-the-by it was not a hall, but the Sessions-house, the audience being seated in the body of the Court and the entertainers appearing on the bench. The Court was like an ice-safe, and my fingers were so cold I could not properly play the piano, and had to apologise for my extra defective execution. I have frequently made my appearance at the Sessions under the above circumstances.

At Cardiff I have always appeared in the Court-house, and a splendid audience I always had. If I remember rightly, the chief seats were in the prisoners' dock, which, [of course, commanded the best view of the entertainers' bench. I knew there was always a rush for the dock—I mean on the nights when my father and I were there; not when the proper judge was there, of course. It seems strange that people should pay for the privilege of being accommodated with a seat in the dock. I ought to mention that the granting of the Court-house for the purpose of entertainments was unusual. It was a favour extended towards well-known lecturers only.

It would be quite impossible, in a small book like this, to describe all the extraordinary incidents which I have encountered while fulfilling my engagements (before I went on the stage, of course) at the various country institutions. By institutions I refer to the societies which were formed all over the United Kingdom chiefly for the benefit of the better-class working men and women, and the popularity of which is on the wane, owing to the prevalence of free libraries, penny readings, and amateur concerts.

Some of these institutions, which provide reading and writing rooms, debating classes, educational classes, and a room or rooms for concerts and lectures, etc., can boast a really magnificent building—for an institution. I have most pleasant recollections of the Leeds Mechanics' Institution, the Bradford, the Edinburgh, Plymouth, &c.; for they possessed splendid halls for acoustics, a good platform, a capital grand piano (most welcome to me), always a crowded audience (most welcome to everybody), and they refrained from commencing the proceedings—at all events when I gave my humorous recitals—with prayer. Oh yes, gentle reader, my comic recitals have frequently been commenced with prayer—nearly always at the Young Men's Christian Literary Institutions. Sometimes, in addition, there would be a short sermon.

I have a distinct recollection of an amiable curate, at the conclusion of one of my country engagements, rising to propose a vote of thanks to me. He was most flattering and kind in his observations, and being a little unorthodox (for a country village), impressed upon the audience that there was "no sin in a genuine hearty laugh." He meant well, no doubt; but as the audience had not laughed in the least throughout my recital, I thought the curate's remark rather superfluous.

Some fifteen or sixteen years ago I was engaged to give a short entertainment, for a still shorter fee, at some schoolrooms connected with a church in Camden Town. The rooms were in a small back street adjacent to the High Street. The festivities consisted of a spread of tea and what Mr. W. S. Gilbert calls "the rollicking bun and the gay Sally Lunn," interspersed with conversation, songs by amateurs, homely advice by the vicar, and a few comic songs—I beg pardon, I should say "humorous ditties"—by myself.

The rooms were crowded with the poorer parishioners, who ought, each Sunday, to have attended the church, but did not as a matter of fact. Most of the husbands could not come to the entertainment, for reasons best known to themselves, but their wives and babies did. I never sang to so many women and babies before or since. I like an audience consisting of ladies: they do not make such a visible sign of enjoyment as do the sterner sex, but they have a much keener appreciation of satire, music, and humour. But ladies without babies and with babies are totally different people. The moment a baby makes its presence known to an audience it is all up with the entertainer; competition is useless, and he may as well retire from the platform.

On this occasion there were fifty babies and general chaos. The mothers became anxious and the audience demoralised. At last it was my turn to sing. I was about to step on to platform, when the vicar said to me, " Mr. Grossmith—one moment, please. I am most desirous that these poor folk should enjoy themselves, and I do not wish to inflict upon them anything approaching a sermon. At the same time I want most particularly to impress upon them the necessity of their attending church occasionally. Now I thought you might drop them a little reminder about the non-observance of the Sabbath, which is, unfortunately, characteristic of them."

" Do you seriously want me to do that?" I asked.

" Certainly," he replied. " It would appear less like a sermon, and they might take it better from you than from me."

" You had better do it yourself," I said; "for I have no doubt if I did it they would put it down as part of the comic entertainment, and it would be received with roars of laughter."

" Ah! that would never do," said the vicar. " Very well, Mr. Grossmith, I will act upon your suggestion and do it myself."

The vicar proceeded with a rather lengthy

serious speech, the peroration of which was much like the following :

"In conclusion, my friends, no excuse can be accepted for your not coming occasionally to church. I hear too often from you that you cannot leave your babies. Mrs. Brown says she cannot leave hers, and Mrs. Jones tells me she cannot leave hers, and so it goes on. But you can befriend each other. Mrs. Brown can mind her own babies as well as Mrs. Jones's for one Sunday, and Mrs. Jones can do the same for Mrs. Brown the following Sunday. You would then be able to come once a fortnight at all events. It is a duty that devolves upon you, and a duty you must, at all hazards, perform. Remember this, my friends—you *must* try and come to church. Mr. Grossmith will now sing '*I am so Volatile.*'"

One night there was a break-down on the railway line, and my father and myself never arrived in the town until twenty past eight, although we should have commenced at eight punctually. We dressed in the cab, which flew along like a fire-engine. Suddenly we espied a building lighted up, and a large crowd coming out. My father pushed his head out of the window and shouted frantically to the crowd, "Go back! Go back! It's all right. Grossmith is here. We have arrived. Go back!" Unfortunately it was not our audience, but a congregation leaving a Methodist Chapel.

In 1876 Miss Florence Marryat, the novelist and daughter of the celebrated Capt. Marryat, talked over a joint entertainment. It was quite apparent that the literary institutions were "not what they were." Their fees, like their engagements, were rapidly decreasing. Miss Marryat and I thought out a programme, and determined to appeal more generally to the public. I append one of the programmes:

PROGRAMME
OF
"ENTRE NOUS."

PROLOGUE...Spoken by FLORENCE MARRYAT,
and interrupted by GEO. GROSSMITH, JUN.

HUMOROUS MUSICAL SCENA... "On the Sands" ... *Grossmith*.
GEO. GROSSMITH, JUN.

COSTUME RECITAL... "Joan of Arc in Prison"... *James Albery*.
FLORENCE MARRYAT.
(With the Scena by LINDSAY SLOPER.)

HUMOROUS MUSICAL SCENA..."A Cold Collation"...*Grossmith*.
GEO. GROSSMITH, JUN.

COSTUME RECITAL..." The Grandmother" ... ... *Tennyson*.
FLORENCE MARRYAT.

HISTORICAL MEDLEY..." Richard Cœur-de-Léon "...*E. Draper*.

INTERVAL OF THREE MINUTES.

To conclude with a Satirical Musical Sketch, entitled

"CUPS AND SAUCERS."

(Written and Composed expressly by GEO. GROSSMITH, Jun.)

MRS. EMILY NANKEEN WORCESTER
(A China Maniac) ... FLORENCE MARRYAT.

GENERAL DEELAH
(Another) ... ... ... GEO. GROSSMITH, JUN.

The above is the last joint entertainment I ever gave, except with my father, and I only fulfilled one or two more with him.

"Cups and Saucers" was afterwards played before *H.M.S. Pinafore*, at the Opera Comique, for about 500 nights. It is still played a great deal by amateurs all over the country, both with and without my permission. This entertainment with Miss Marryat was more of an artistic success than a financial one. Sometimes we did very well, and sometimes we did not. In Scotland we always had crowded rooms; but at the Antient Concert Rooms, Dublin, we played a whole month, the majority of the time to half-full rooms. I enjoyed the month in Dublin, for all that. The people were most hospitable; and so Florence Marryat, her companion (Miss Glover), Mr. George Dolby, and myself managed to enjoy ourselves. Henry Irving was in Dublin at the time, and, as I had the privilege of being an old friend of his, I naturally came in for all his parties; and Irving is a prince of hosts.

Florence Marryat, in her excellent book *Tom Tiddler's Ground*, has regaled her readers with several stories about me; so I am going to have my revenge. She is a great believer in spiritualism, and on one occasion, in Dublin, she persuaded me to sit at a table with her. The table began to tilt, rap, creak, and move; and it is not in my province to attempt to explain the marvellous phenomena. My explanation would be too simple to be scientific. The conditions, however, are, that if the table tilts three times in answer to a question, it means "Yes," and if only once "No." Florence Marryat informed me—and I have no reason to doubt her word—that a gentleman, with a name something like "Sticks," was endeavouring to communicate with her through the table. It appears that poor "Sticks" had left this world through an excess of stimulants. Two questions were asked by Miss Marryat, and replied to by "Sticks." At last Mr. "Sticks" condescended, with three tilts, to imply that he would answer my questions. Miss Marryat begged that I would not be irreverent; and I argued that if I were, I presumed "Sticks" would treat me with contempt.

I said to the table: "Mr. Sticks, I wish to ask you a few questions?"

[By-the-by, I believe he was a "Colonel Sticks." It is of little consequence now in this story; but it was at the time, for spirits, like human beings, are most particular about being addressed by their proper titles.]

In reply to my question, "Sticks" oscillated the table violently, which, I was informed, meant agitation on his part. Florence Marryat told me the poor chap was in purgatory.

I said: "Sticks, I believe you died of drink?" Three decisive tilts of the table.

"Now, Mr. Sticks," I asked, "is it possible to take too much drink in purgatory?"

The table was seized with convulsions, and wriggled and oscillated to a corner of the room. When it was quiet, I said:

"Mr. Sticks, do not think I mean to be disrespectful; but are you drunk now?"

Then came three solemn but distinct tilts.

Florence Marryat considered I was most discourteous to poor "Sticks," and has never since sat with me at a table, except for lunch or dinner.

A sudden illness of Miss Marryat was, on one occasion, the cause of an unrehearsed, but withal very successful, entertainment.

Miss Marryat and I were announced to appear at the Town Hall, Cardiff, in our entertainment, " Entre Nous." I copy the following from a Cardiff paper of February 1st, 1877 :

"MR. GEO. GROSSMITH, JUN., AT THE TOWN HALL, CARDIFF.—Between you and me, gentle reader, or, as the advertisements have had it so prominently of late, *entre nous*, there was no ' Entre Nous ' at the Assembly Rooms, Cardiff, last night. At the last moment it was announced that Miss Florence Marryat was incapacitated by a serious illness from taking her part in the promised performance. A capital audience had been drawn to the Town Hall, a large number of whom were, doubtless, attracted by the expectation of seeing this talented authoress and most gifted *artiste*. It is, however, only due to them to say that they bore their disappointment kindly, and, with only one exception, the whole of the audience—although the promoters of the entertainment offered to return their money at the doors—remained to witness the single-handed entertainment provided by Mr. George Grossmith, jun. And it was well for them they did so, for they enjoyed a treat which must have made even Miss Marryat's absence almost appear in the light of a blessing. At the last moment, whilst the audience were grimly reading the announcement of that lady's sudden illness, at the time when consternation was reigning in the bosom of those enterprising *entrepreneurs*, Messrs. Thompson and Shackell, and whilst Mr. George Grossmith, jun., was shivering in his shoes with timidity at the thought of the cool reception which, in his bereaved condition, he was likely to obtain, a sudden and a happy thought flashed across the mind of one of his friends. 'Why not get Courtenay Clarke* to give you a lift, my boy?' suggested one of the bystanders. 'I scarcely dare ask him,' replied the desponding entertainer. 'Oh, but he was one of your father's warmest friends,' rejoined the speaker; 'and his good nature is only equalled by his marvellous comic power. Anyhow, you can try it, for I see that he and Colonel Page have just entered the room.' And so the attempt upon Mr. Clarke's good nature was made; and, fortunately, it was successful. There was a mysterious whispering between Mr. Shackell and the intended victim. Then the pair retired to the ante-room, and their arguments were addressed to Mr. Clarke's kindly feeling of friendship, which resulted in the appearance on the platform, very shortly afterwards, of the clever young entertainer, escorted by Mr. Clarke, who took the chair. In a speech of inimitable humour, he explained and apologised for the absence of Miss Marryat, and introduced, with words of encouragement, the younger Grossmith. Of this gentleman's performance it is scarcely necessary to speak in detail. It is the very essence of refined musical comedy."

* Mr. Courtenay C. Clarke was a resident at Cardiff, who generally entertained my father and myself on our professional visits. He became a great friend of mine, and he was a most talented amateur reciter and *raconteur*. I last saw him about two years ago, when he and Colonel C. Page, of Cardiff (also an intimate friend of mine), supped with me at the Garrick.

Here follow twenty-eight lines of such a flattering description that my modesty (forgive me, gentle reader) will not permit of my reproducing them. The notice continues thus:

"Gratified, however, as everybody was with Mr. Grossmith's performance, the real 'fun of the fair' commenced when Mr. Courtenay Clarke essayed his wonderful reminiscences of Mr. Grossmith the elder. With marvellous fidelity, Mr. Clarke has caught the very trick of voice and manner which constitute the chiefest charm of that mellow humorist. One could almost imagine one was in Mr. Grossmith's company whilst listening to Mr. Clarke's side-splitting imitations. The delicate little side-hits, and exposition of social and personal foibles, added life to the sketch; so that the audience were constrained to laugh at George Grossmith himself, as well as at the delightful comic "bits" which constitute his well-known entertainment. . . . Altogether, we can honestly say that a better or more acceptable entertainment than was given at the Town Hall last night has seldom been witnessed in Cardiff."

Perhaps the most amusing incident that ever occurred to Florence Marryat and myself was at the time we were giving a Saturday night's entertainment at a large hall to a popular audience at Glasgow. A brusque and brawny Scotchman was the caretaker, or hall-porter. I sought him out and informed him that there was neither towel nor soap in either of the dressing-rooms.

He firmly told me that I must find my own

towel and soap, as it did not answer his purpose to do so.

I asked what he meant.

He said that the entertainers generally stole the soap and towels afterwards.

There was no attempt to wrap up the accusation. He called a spade a spade, without doubt. I was very indignant, and said: "Do you dare to insinuate that a lady like Florence Marryat, a well-known novelist, would steal your penn'orth of soap and fourpenny towel?"

He replied: "I don't know anything about Miss Marryat, and I don't care. All I know is, you entertainers always do walk off with my soap and towels, and I'll ha' no more of it."

## CHAPTER VI.

### Gilbert and Sullivan.

"Then I can hum a fugue, of which I've heard the music's *din afore*,
And whistle all the airs from that infernal nonsense, *Pinafore*."
*The Pirates of Penzance.*

I PLAYED in comparatively few amateur theatrical performances—half a dozen, at the outside. I played John Chodd, jun., in *Society*, at the old Gallery of Illustration, in 1868; and, singularly enough, one of my critics was Mr. W. S. Gilbert, who, under the heading of "The Theatrical Lounger," in *The Illustrated Times*, said: "Mr. Grossmith has comic powers of no mean order; and his idea of John Chodd, carefully modelled on Mr. Clarke, had, nevertheless, an amusing originality of its own." The after-piece was a burlesque on *No Thoroughfare*, written by my father, in which I danced and sang more than I acted. This performance was repeated once.

I then essayed the part of Paul Pry, in Poole's comedy of that name, at the Gallery of Illustration, in 1870, and played in the after-piece a burlesque of which I was part author. These performances went off very well, and we were very much complimented (as all amateurs are), and declared our attempts to have eclipsed our neighbours (as all amateurs do). But such a thought as going on the stage never entered my head for a moment; I refused several offers, including a good one from Mr. E. P. Hingston to appear in the comic opera *La Branche Cassée*, at the Opéra Comique, the very theatre at which I was destined to make my *début*.

After entertaining all over the country for seven years, I made a rather important discovery; viz., that my income was as rapidly *de*creasing each year as my family and household expenses were *in*creasing. I disliked being away so long from London; for there is nothing so valuable to any public singer or actor as the constant appearance of his name in the entertainments or theatrical columns of the metropolitan daily papers.

I had begun my autumn and winter tour with my father for 1877–8, when, in the November of 1877, I received the following letter:

"Beefsteak Club,
"King William Street, W.C.
"Tuesday Night.

"Dear Mr. Grossmith,—Are you inclined to go on the stage for a time? There is a part in the new piece I am doing with Gilbert which I think you would play admirably. I can't find a good man for it. Let me have a line, or come to 9 Albert Mansions to-morrow after 4, or Thursday before 2.30.

"Yours sincerely,
"Arthur Sullivan."

The great compliment which I considered the letter conveyed filled me with more delight than I ever could express. I think I read the letter over twenty times. I was not thinking of the offer of the engagement, for I was immediately under the impression that I should decline it. My father never had a good opinion of my amateur acting, and I valued his judgment so highly that his opinion was in a great measure shared by me.

Arthur Sullivan had only heard me sing once, after a dinner party, and it was evident, from his letter, I had created some sound impression; hence my extreme delight at his offer. I remember, after the said party, Sir Arthur (he was then Mr.) kindly asked me back to his rooms, with a few other friends, including Alfred Cellier, the composer, and Arthur Cecil, to whom I was (and still am) much indebted for the most valuable hints he had from time to time given me respecting the style of sketch and song suitable for "smart" drawing-room work, and who had taken great interest in me. At Sullivan's, that evening, we all sang, played, and chatted till an early hour in the morning; and I, as a comparatively "new" man, was especially "drawn out."

Following Arthur Sullivan's letter, with its complimentary offer, came a long one from Arthur Cecil (who, it appears, had suggested my name to Sullivan), pointing out the *pros* and *cons*, with an additional "summing up" of both, worthy of a judge—and a good judge, too.

Cecil told me afterwards that Sullivan and he were both writing letters at the Beefsteak, when the former said, "I can't find a fellow for this opera."

Arthur Cecil said, "I wonder if Grossmith——"

Before the sentence was completed, Arthur Sullivan said, "The very man!"

I was then communicated with. I am much indebted to these two Arthurs. I reverence the name of Arthur; and if ever I am blessed with another son—— But there! as they say in novels, "I am digressing."

Then came a week of awful anxiety. Should I cancel the provincial engagements which I had already made, and which were, of course, a certainty, in favour of a new venture, which was not? My father said, "Not." He did not think I had voice enough. Arthur Sullivan, however, thought I had. I went to consult him, and he struck the D (fourth line in treble clef, if you please), and said, "Sing it out as loud as you can." I did. Sullivan looked up, with a most humorous expression on his face—even his eye-glass seemed to smile—and he simply said, "Beautiful!" Sullivan then sang, "My name is John Wellington Wells," and said, "You can do that?"

I replied, "Yes; I think I can do that."

"Very well," said Sir Arthur, "if you can do that, you can do the rest."

Then off I went to W. S. Gilbert, at Bolton Gardens, to see what the part itself was like. Mr. Gilbert was very kind, and seemed pleased that I meditated accepting the engagement. [A few months beforehand I had played the Judge, in *Trial by Jury*, at the Hall in Archer Street, Bayswater, and the rehearsals were conducted by Mr. Gilbert, who himself coached me for the first time.] Gilbert read me the opening speech of J. W. Wells, with reference to the sale, "Penny curses," &c., with which, of course, I was much amused, and said he had not completed the second act yet; but the part of Wells had developed into greater prominence than was at first anticipated. I saw that the part would suit me excellently, but I said to Mr. Gilbert, "For the part of a Magician I should have thought you required a fine man with a fine voice."

I can still see Gilbert's humorous expression as he replied, "No; that is just what we don't want."

I then went to Mr. R. D'Oyly Carte, who had hit upon the idea of comic opera, by English author and composer, and interpreted by English artists, and who formed the Comedy Opera Company Limited, for the purpose of starting the venture at the Opéra Comique. I asked Carte if he could give me a day or two to think of it. The request was granted, apparently to oblige me; but I imagined, from his look, that D'Oyly Carte also required a day or two to think of it.

I afterwards learned that the directors of the Comedy Opera Company, to a man, were adverse to my engagement. One of them sent the following telegram to Carte: "Whatever you do, don't engage Grossmith." I myself personally was being tossed on the terrible billows of indecision. I had a certain amount of confidence in myself, but thought that if the piece failed — and the Opéra Comique had been an unlucky theatre — I should practically be thrown on my beam ends, having cancelled all my provincial engagements; and they were not many.

I thought, however, that the advertisement of being associated with W. S. Gilbert and Arthur Sullivan would be invaluable; and, in spite of the entreaties of all my friends, I decided to write and accept the engagement. I informed my father of my decision, and he did not hesitate to express his disappointment, not to say disapproval. To my great joy and relief, I received the following letter from Mrs. Howard Paul, whose opinion on all professional matters I esteemed most highly, and who had always given me so much encouragement:

*Private.*]  "17 The Avenue,
"Bedford Park,
"Turnham Green.

"My dear Brother George,—May I claim the privilege of an old friend, and be impertinent enough to make a suggestion and give my opinion?—which is as follows: First, that, under any circumstances, and at some sacrifice, you do not fail to accept the part of the 'Magician' in Gilbert and Sullivan's new play. It is a splendid part—better than you think, I fancy—and the 'patter song' is great in its way. Make your time suit them, or theirs suit you, if possible. I have sacrificed a week's business engagements. This is only a hint to you. I think, if you will arrange, it will be a new and *magnificent introduction* for you, and be of very great service afterwards. I'm sure the part will suit you exactly. Don't think me impertinent in writing this; but I want to see your name in the cast. If I have any influence with you, now's the time to prove it. . . . I suppose you know Mr. Barrington and self play

in the aforesaid piece. Write me per return, and, with love to you all, believe me,
"Yours affectionately,
"Isabella Howard Paul."

This was a great comfort to me—in fact, to all of us. I wrote Mrs. Howard Paul that I had decided to take the engagement; and on the 5th November, 1877, she, Barrington and myself, and a few others, celebrated the event in the back garden at Bedford Park with a display of fireworks.

Messrs. Gilbert, Sullivan, and Carte backed up the engagement with me, and the directors, though in the majority, were, happily for me, defeated.

Then came the business part of the matter with D'Oyly Carte, which was amusing. As I had sacrificed my country engagements, I wished Carte to guarantee me a month's salary. That request he acceded to, but not to the amount of salary I required. He was instructed "only to go to a certain amount," which happened to be three guineas a week less than I asked for. The discussion, such as it was, was quite pleasant, as, in fact, all my future negotiations with him were destined to be. I have been associated with Mr. D'Oyly Carte for over ten years now, and am pleased to say I have never had anything approaching a disagreeable word with him.

I said to Carte: "Look at the risk I am running. If I fail, I don't believe the Young Men's Christian Associations will ever engage me again, because I have appeared on the stage, and my reputation as comic singer to religious communities will be lost for ever."

Carte said, "Well, I dare say I can make that all right." Then a sudden idea occurred to him. "Come and have some oysters."

I did!! I shall ever regret it! A lunch off oysters and most excellent Steinberg Cabinet infused a liberality into my nature for which I shall never forgive myself. Carte again broached the subject—*after lunch*—of the salary; and in the end, with a cheerful smile, I waived the extra three guineas a week.

I calculate that, irrespective of all accumulative interest, that lunch cost me, up till now, about £1,800.

One dark night in that very November I fulfilled my last provincial institution engagement (at Dudley), and went back to stay the night, or what was left of it, at the Guest Hospital, with Dr. Orwin, my old schoolfellow, with whom I had the pugilistic encounter at the preparatory school on Haverstock Hill. He called me up at five o'clock the next morning, which was, if possible, darker than the night before, and packed me off to London to attend my first rehearsal, which was held in the refreshment saloon (without refreshments) at the Opéra Comique.

The course adopted with reference to the Gilbert and Sullivan rehearsals is as follows: The music is always taken first. The principal singers and the ladies and gentlemen of the chorus are seated in a semi-circle on the stage. A cottage piano is in the middle, and we are rehearsed as an ordinary choir would be. Sir Arthur Sullivan usually first composes the difficult choruses, especially the finale to the first act—an elaborate score.

The quartettes and trios arrive next, and the duets and songs last.

I have sometimes only received the tunes of my songs the week before production. The song in the second act of *Princess Ida* was re-written, and I only got the music two nights before the performance. The difficulty then was, not in learning the new tune, but in *un*learning the old one.

The greatest interest is evinced by us all as the new vocal numbers arrive. Sir Arthur Sullivan will arrive hurriedly, with a batch of MSS. under his arm, and announce the fact that there is something new. He takes his seat at the piano and plays over the new number. The vocal parts are written in, but no accompaniment.

Mr. François Cellier listens and watches; and how he can remember for future rehearsal, as he does, the elaborate accompaniments and symphonies, with the correct harmonies, &c., from simply hearing Sir Arthur play the pieces over a few times, is to me astonishing.

Mr. Gilbert will attend all these musical rehearsals: he takes mental notes of the style of composition, time, rhythm, everything, and goes home and invents his groups and business. For every piece he has small stages constructed —exact models of the Savoy Theatre—with set scenes. The characters are represented by little bricks of various colours, to distinguish chorus from principals, and ladies from gentlemen. Many a time he has shown me some future intended grouping, entrance, or general effect; and I must say it has been most interesting. No expense is spared to get the requisite accuracy; and I believe the little model of a ship, for the recent revival of *H.M.S. Pinafore*, cost £60.

It is well known that Mr. Gilbert is an extremely strict man, and on all matters of stage business his word is law. All the arrangements of colours and the original groupings, with which the frequenters of the Savoy are so well acquainted, are by him.

Sir Arthur Sullivan is also very exact with reference to the rendering of the music; and it is perfectly understood between author and composer that no business should be introduced by the former into the chorus so as to interfere with a proper performance of the music.

For example, in the original rehearsals of *The Mikado*, Mr. Gilbert arranged a group of the chorus to "bow down" to his Majesty as he entered, with their backs to the audience. Sir Arthur Sullivan came down, and, the moment he saw this, said that the voices could not be well heard from the front, as the faces of the singers were turned towards the back of the stage. Mr. Gilbert immediately altered the business; and as his powers of invention are apparently unlimited, the present effective grouping in a semi-circle on the right-hand side and back of the stage was substituted.

I have said that Sir Arthur Sullivan is strict with the music. Every member of the chorus has to sing the exact note set down for him or her; and often, in the midst of the rehearsal of a full chorus *double-forte* we have been pulled up because a careless gentleman has sung a semi-quaver instead of a demi-semi-quaver, or one of the cousins, sisters, or aunts has failed to dot a crotchet.

One of the most prominent and popular members of our company was remarkably quick in picking up the music by ear—a method of learning music by no means advisable. One day he was singing a solo allotted to him which he had learned in the way mentioned, and he occasionally sang (let us say) two even crotchets instead of one dotted and a quaver, and he made one or two slight deviations from the melody. Sullivan listened, with a most amused expression, and, at the conclusion, said: "Bravo! that is really a very good tune of yours—capital! And now, if you have no objection, I will trouble you to sing mine."

The music is generally given to us before the piece is read by Mr. Gilbert; so we are often in complete darkness as to the meaning of the words we are singing. In the opera of *Princess Ida* we were rehearsing the whole of the concerted music of the first act. My song, "I can't think why," sung by King Gama, was not composed, and the whole of my share in the rehearsals was the following three bars and a half of recitative:

"*King Gama* (recitative): Must we till then in prison cell be thrust?

"*Hildebrand:* You must.

"*King Gama:* This seems unnecessarily severe."

At one of the rehearsals, after singing this

trifling bit of recitative, I addressed the composer and said:

"Could you tell me, Sir Arthur, what the words, 'This seems unnecessarily severe,' have reference to?"

Sir Arthur Sullivan replied:

"Because you are to be detained in prison, of course."

I replied: "Thank you. I thought they had reference to my having been detained here three hours a day for the past fortnight to sing them."

The result was, that Sir Arthur liberated me from the remainder of the first act rehearsals; and as I had not to put in an appearance in the second act, and had only one unwritten song in the third, I had, for a wonder, a pretty easy time of it.

The musical rehearsals are child's play in comparison with the stage rehearsals. Mr. Gilbert is a perfect autocrat, insisting that his words should be delivered, even to an inflection of the voice, as he dictates. He will stand on the stage beside the actor or actress, and repeat the words with appropriate action over and over again, until they are delivered as he desires them to be. In some instances, of course, he allows a little license, but very little.

He has great patience at times; and, indeed, he needs it, for occasionally one or other of the company, through inaccurate ear or other cause, will not catch the proper action or inflection. From the beginning it has been the custom, if possible, to allot some small part to a member of the chorus. The girls have nearly always benefited by the chance, and some have risen to the foremost ranks. The men are not so fortunate, I regret to say. They do not seem to be so quick. Gilbert has nearly been driven frantic (and so have the onlookers for the matter of that) because a sentence has been repeated with a false accent.

The following sketch, founded on fact, is an example of what I mean:

Suppose Mr. Snooks has been promoted from the chorus, and allotted a very small part, on account of his suitable voice, slimness, stoutness, gigantic proportions, or the reverse. He has one line—let us say, *The King is in the counting-house.* The first thing Mr. Snooks does when his cue arrives is to make the most of his opportunity by entering with a comic slow walk, which he has evidently been studying for the past few days in front of a looking-glass. The walk is the conventional one indulged in by the big Mask in a pantomime.

*Mr. Gilbert:* Please don't enter like that, Mr. Snooks. We don't want any "comic man" business here.

*Mr. Snooks:* I beg your pardon, sir; I thought you meant the part to be funny.

*Mr. Gilbert:* Yes, so I do; but I don't want you to *tell* the audience you're the funny man. They'll find it out, if you are, quickly enough. Go on, please.

Mr. Snooks enters again with a rapid and sharp catch-the-six-thirteen-Liverpool-street-local-train kind of walk.

*Mr. Gilbert:* No, no, no, Mr. Snooks. This is not a "walking gentleman's" part. As it is only a short one, there is no necessity to hurry through it like that.  Enter like this.

Mr. Gilbert proceeds to exemplify what he requires, and after a trial or two Mr. Snooks gets it nearly right.

*Mr. Gilbert* (encouragingly): That'll do capitally.  Go on, please.

*Mr. Snooks:* The King is in the counting-*house*.

*Mr. Gilbert:* No, no, Mr. Snooks; he is nothing of the sort.  He is in the *counting*-house.

*Mr. Snooks:* The King is in the counting-*house*.

*Mr. Gilbert* (very politely): I am afraid I have not made myself understood.  It is not counting-*house*, but *counting*-house.  Do you understand me?

*Mr. Snooks:* Yes, sir.

*Mr. Gilbert:* Very well; try again, please.

*Mr. Snooks:* The King is in the counting-*house*.

*Mr. Gilbert* (still politely): Mr. Snooks, don't you appreciate the difference between the accent on "counting" and the accent on "house"?  I want the accent on "counting"—*counting*-house.  Surely you have never heard it pronounced in any other way?  Try again, and *please* pay attention.

*Mr. Snooks* (getting rather nervous): The King is in the counting-HOUSE!

Mr. Gilbert twitches his right whisker, and takes a few paces up and down the front of the stage.  Eventually he comes to a standstill, and calmly addresses Mr. Snooks:

"It is my desire to assist you as far as I possibly can, but I *must* have that sentence spoken properly.  I would willingly cut it out altogether; but as it is essential to the story, that course is impossible. If you cannot speak it with the right accent, I shall be reluctantly compelled to give the words to someone else who *can*. Go back, please, and *think* before you speak."

*Mr. Snooks* (endeavouring to think he is "thinking"): The King (pause) is (pause) IN the . . . (very long pause) *counting* . . . (with a violent effort) HOUSE !!!

*Mr. Gilbert* (bottling up his fury): We won't bother about your scene now, Mr. Snooks. Get on with the next. Grossmith! Grossmith!! (To Seymour, the stage manager): Where's Mr. Grossmith?

*Mr. Grossmith* (a very small man, with a still smaller voice): Here I am.

*Mr. Gilbert:* Oh! there you are. I'm sorry to have kept you waiting. We'll go on with your scene. Do you want to try your song?

*Mr. Grossmith:* Not unless you want to hear it!

*Mr. Gilbert:* No; I don't want to hear it. (Roars of laughter from the company.) Do you?

*Mr. Grossmith:* No!

Good humour prevails, and the rehearsal proceeds. At its termination Mr. Gilbert approaches Mr. Snooks, who is absolutely wretched in the corner.

*Mr. Gilbert* (privately to Mr. Snooks): Don't worry yourself about that. Go home, and think it over. It will be all right to-morrow.

On the morrow, perhaps, it is *not* all right; but Mr. Gilbert will pass it over, and by dint of perseverance (which is, of course, appreciated), and the chaffing he gets from his fellow-choristers at the theatre, and the bullying from his wife at home, Mr. Snooks, in the course of a week, gets it actually right; but the word is always pronounced to the end with a certain amount of doubt.

The performer frequently gets the credit which is due to Mr. Gilbert, and to him absolutely. As a rule, the little midshipmite in *H.M.S. Pinafore* is supposed to be a perfect genius. There have been scores of midshipmites in town and "on tour," but they are all geniuses.

Some, of course, are naturally clever, and I should be grieved to disparage any child; but if admiration, cheers, and applause on the stage are at all times dangerous to the mind of man, what must be the effect on children!

A little boy, with a pretty voice, who played in the performance of the *Pirates of Penzance* by children, came to me some time back in despair. His vanity had been touched by the approbation of the public, and his eyes fascinated by the glare of the footlights and limelights. They were all he thought of. His voice had gone, or, to be more accurate, had cracked. He was too old to act as a child, and too young to act as a man; and he "pooh-poohed" any idea of an ordinary situation. All the credit of his success his friends attributed to his own talent, and not to his stage manager.

It is such a case as this, and this only, that induces me to say that I have seen Mr. Gilbert instruct a little boy in the part of the midshipmite for an hour or so at a time, simply how to walk across the stage. The boy has been absolutely stupid even for his age; but has been selected because he happened to be smaller than the others who had come up for competition. Through constant drilling the child developed into a mechanical toy, and received the approbation of the generous public, as if he merited it instead of his tutor, when he had no more done so than the little canary who walks the tight-rope on a barrow, fires a gun, or drives a tandem drawn by a couple of sparrows.

One of these little lads, besides his wages, received extra presents of shillings and half-crowns that in the course of a week amounted, most likely, to the limited salary given to the chorus man who had devoted the greater part of his life to his vocation, and who had a wife and large family to support out of it.

*Apropos* of the chorus, they are picked from hundreds who first sing before Mr. D'Oyly Carte on approval. They generally have some daily occupation or situation. Some of them sing and act so well in the groups that they have been retained from the very commencement of the operas.

When *Iolanthe* was produced, Gilbert decided that the peers should all have the upper lip shaven, and wear "mutton-chop" whiskers, and a little tuft under the lower lip. They were also to wear wigs bald at the top of the head. The effect was ultimately most successful; but there was a semblance of a "strike" beforehand, owing to the objection of some of the gentlemen to shave off the moustache.

These were called, for the purpose of giving their reasons for objecting to comply with the order. Some of the excuses were most amusing. One said he was a town traveller; and if he took off his moustache, he would look so young that shopowners would not listen to him. Another said he was a "spirit leveller," and it was most unusual (I am not sure he did not say unprecedented) for a "spirit leveller" *not* to have a moustache. The excuse for another gentlemen was, that he was paying his addresses to a young lady who was not much impressed with his personal appearance; and if he took off his moustache, his hopes would be completely blighted. In the end, however, they all consented to obliterate the ornament, with the exception of one, who absolutely declined. In his case the moustache stayed on, but he did not.

I never remember, before the Gilbert and Sullivan operas, to have seen an entire chorus shaved. The peers looked wonderfully characteristic when they first appeared over the bridge, and their entrance brought down the house. Again, what could be more effective than the shaven faces in *The Mikado?*

The most amusing incident with regard to shaving was during the run of *Ruddygore*. A rather good-looking young fellow, a new comer, was requested to shave (the others being already shaven) a fortnight before the production of the piece, in order that his photograph in costume might be taken by Messrs. Barraud. The portraits that hung in the picture gallery of Sir

Ruthven Murgatroyd were painted from the photographs previously taken of all the chorus gentlemen. This new recruit, whom we will call Mr. X., was a concert singer, who, like many others, finding that "concert singing is not what it was," accepted the offer made to him to join the ranks of the Savoyards as a chorister, and make sure of a certain income. Mr. D'Oyly Carte met him one day, and said:

"Have you been to Barraud's, Mr. X.?"

"No, sir; I go to-morrow morning. I have shaved."

"So I observe," said Carte.

Two days after, Carte saw him with his moustache on again; but, taking no particular notice, said:

"Let me see, have you been to Barraud's?"

Mr. X. said: "Yes, sir; I went yesterday."

D'Oyly Carte thought it seemed rather odd, for he made sure he had seen Mr. X. two days previously without the moustache. Now he had a full-grown one, with the regular platform singer's waxed ends.

D'Oyly Carte, being a busy man, walked away, and was soon thinking of other matters.

The first dress rehearsal took place, and Mr. X. had no moustache. Mr. Carte met him the next day in the street, and, lo and behold! there was the moustache on again. Actors are frequently in the habit of "soaping" down their moustaches; but such a one as Mr. X. supported could not be soaped down. Carte was so puzzled that he said to Mr. X.:

"I thought you had shaved your moustache?"

Mr. X. replied: "So I have, sir; but when

I sing at concerts, or 'do' Bond Street, I stick on one for a little while. Nobody would notice it was not my own, and I look so much better with a moustache."

"Do you make yourself up, Mr. Grossmith?"

As this question is so frequently asked of me, I will satisfy the curious by saying that I always do. No one has ever touched my face but myself. I select my own colours, powders, rouges, and try several effects of complexions, before finally deciding on one. I have a little dressing-room to myself—the only one who has at the Savoy. Being short-sighted, I make up with a hand-glass in my left hand. My dressing-table is very high, and I have several bright electric lights thrown on my face. I do not think the painted lines on the face should ever be seen, even from the stalls. I think no make-up should be detected from the front, and I have no hesitation in saying that the ghastly white faces, pink cheeks, and scarlet lips indulged in, even by the ladies of our theatre, are simply hideous.

Mr. Barrington has often come into my room just as I am going on the stage, and chaffingly said, "Why don't you make up?" I regard this rather as a compliment than otherwise.

I want to look like a First Lord, a fleshly poet, Major-General, or Japanese, not to *show* how I look like one.

The walls of my dressing-room are covered with prints, engravings, and sketches, of no particular value, but of interest to myself and many who visit me.

A capital pen-and-ink sketch, from memory, by Mr. Heather Bigg, of Corney Grain and myself playing a duet on the piano, amuses those who see it. A slight sketch by Frank Holl, R.A. (a great and esteemed friend of mine), of myself, fishing in the daytime and doing the Lord Chancellor's dance at night, is, of course, interesting.

There is also a water-colour sketch of myself in the costume of King Gama, *minus* the heavy cloak and wig, and the tunic preserved by a lawn-tennis jacket. I used to sit in this comfortable way during a long wait of one hour and forty minutes; and my appearance so tickled the fancy of Viscount Hardinge that he painted his impression of it, and sent it to me.

There is also an admirable sketch, by Alfred Bryan, of John Parry; a signed photograph of Mrs. Howard Paul; full-page drawings in the *Graphic*, &c., from my brother's pictures exhibited in the Royal Academy; some old playbills, in which my uncle figures prominently; clever sketches of singers, by Harper Pennington; and, what is more useful than any of the above, a comfortable couch, on which I can throw myself after having been encored two or three times in some extravagant dance.

The rules behind the scenes at the Savoy are very strict. No visitors, thank goodness, are allowed to be hanging about the stage or standing at the wings. There are separate staircases for the ladies and gentlemen. We are all a very happy family; jealous feeling and spirit are conspicuous by their absence; and the "understudies" experience no difficulty in getting every help and support, if required, from the principals whose parts are to be played in case of absence or illness.

There are no mashers waiting at the stage-door. Presents and love-letters are few and far between; in fact, during the ten years I have been on the stage I have only received one. I confess I am a little hurt by the notion; but, perhaps it is just as well. The letter referred to was not well worded, and the spelling certainly might have been better. The lady, I am sure, was quite sincere in her expressed adoration of me, and I appreciated her candid confession that she had no prejudice against my "calling"; but the *postscript* was certainly disappointing. It ran thus:

"P.S.—Next Sunday is my Sunday out."

Before engaging anybody at the theatre, Mr. D'Oyly Carte hears them sing, or "tries their voice." It is a standing joke between him and myself that I never kept the appointments made by him to "hear my voice."

At one of our pleasant annual theatre suppers, at which both gentlemen of the orchestra and chorus are present, in returning thanks for having my health proposed, I said I attributed the pleasure of being associated with them to the fact that, in the first instance, I would *not* let Mr. Carte have the opportunity of testing my vocal powers; for, if I had done so, I should never have effected my present engagement.

During D'Oyly Carte's visits to America, Mr. Michael Gunn, the lessee of the Dublin Theatre, and a great friend of both Carte and myself, used to act as our manager.

On one occasion Mr. Gunn had to try the voices of some candidates for the chorus. One gentleman, who called himself Signor Concertini, or some such name, sang all right; but he spoke with an affected broken-English accent, which I have found quite common amongst English foreign singers.

Mr. R. Barker, a kind but rather brusque stage-manager, addressing Signor Concertini, said:

"Look here, my boy, that accent won't do for sailors or pirates. Just give us a little less Mediterranean and a little more Whitechapel."

Mr. Gunn turned to the man and said:

"What nationality are you? You don't sound Italian."

Signor Concertini suddenly dropped his accent, and, addressing Mr. Gunn in a broad Irish brogue, said:

"Sure, Mr. Gunn, I'm from the same country as yourself."

If any of the members of the chorus are absent through illness, they are supposed to bring a doctor's certificate the next day; but their word is usually taken.

One of the chorus gentlemen, a tenor, who had not distinguished himself by any great ability, but deemed his presence of infinite importance, sent a telegram to the stage manager: "Suffering from hoarseness; cannot appear to-night." I ascertained that he had informed several of his colleagues, confidentially, that he was the future Sims Reeves. I must confess, with the exception of the above telegram, I had detected no resemblance to the great tenor.

During the revival of *H.M.S. Pinafore* at the Savoy, I received a dreadful snub from one of the "Marines." The Marines were what is theatrically known as "extra-gentlemen." They are not engaged to sing, and therefore do not hold such a good position as the chorus. If they have voices and can sing, they look forward naturally to promotion. One of them asked me if I would hear him sing the "Ruler of the Queen's Navee." I made an appointment with him to sing at my house. After he finished the song, I said:

"I presume you desire me to recommend you to Mr. Carte for the chorus?"

"Oh no, sir," he replied. "Mr. Carte has heard me, and says I'm not good enough for the chorus; so I thought you could recommend me to him to play *your* parts on tour."

Singers, prima donnas especially, are, I believe, renowned for little airs and graces; but these have little weight with Gilbert and Sullivan. Conventionality is not recognised by them. One of the many Josephines, during the first run of *Pinafore*, objected to standing anywhere but in the centre of the stage, assuring Mr. Gilbert that she had played in Italian opera, and was accustomed to occupy that position and no other.

Gilbert said, most persuasively:

"Oh! but this is *not* Italian opera; this is

only a low burlesque of the worst possible kind."

Gilbert says this sort of thing in such a quiet and serious way that one scarcely knows whether he is joking or not.

During the revival of *The Mikado*, he was directing the dress-rehearsal from the middle of the stalls, as is his wont, and suddenly called out:

"There is a gentleman in the left group not holding his fan correctly."

The stage manager, with his prompt-book and tall hat, immediately appeared on the stage at the left side, and, calling to Mr. Gilbert, said:

"One gentleman is absent through illness, sir."

"Ah!" said Gilbert, perfectly seriously, "that is not the gentleman I am referring to."

Yet another instance. The second act of *The Pirates of Penzance* represents the interior of a ruined abbey by moonlight. Near the end of the play General Stanley's daughters run on to the stage in *peignoir* and with lighted candles. This is the cue for turning up the footlights and boarders.

*Mr. Gilbert* (from the stalls): Mr. Seymour— Mr. Seymour!

*Seymour* (the stage manager, appearing at the wings): Yes, sir.

*Mr. Gilbert*: Don't let them turn the lights on the back cloth!

*Seymour*: We have turned up all the lights, sir.

*Mr. Gilbert*: Then don't do so. As much

light in the front as you like. Candles on the stage have a wonderful effect, I know. They would light up the abbey, no doubt; but even stage candles wouldn't light up the heavens beyond.

A great objection was taken, both by the press and a large section of the public, to the title of *Ruddygore*, and the opera itself was not favourably criticised. About a week after its production, Gilbert turned up at the Savoy and said :

" I propose altering the title of the piece, and calling it *Kensington Gore; or, Not so Good as The Mikado.*"

Gilbert very properly objects to any business being interpolated without his sanction, especially if its sole object is merely to raise a laugh, and thereby stop the action of the piece. In *The Mikado*, Miss Jessie Bond and I were kneeling side by side, with our heads on the floor, and she used to give me a push, and I accordingly rolled completely over. Gilbert asked me if I would mind omitting that action on my part.

I replied :

" Certainly, if you wish it ; but I get an enormous laugh by it."

" So you would if you sat on a pork-pie," replied he.

It is a very easy thing to get a laugh on the stage, and a very difficult thing to sacrifice it. It has amused me intensely when some of the gentlemen who play my parts on the country tour inform me of certain laughs which they get when *they* play. Some of them have even kindly advised me of "new business" which they have inserted.

I quite agree with Mr. Gilbert in reference to the "pork-pie" method of obtaining laughter; and I have often stated that my ambition is, to play in a farce in which there is a bandbox placed carefully on an arm-chair, and that the curtain should finally fall *without* my having sat on the box in question.

I have no intention of dwelling on the incidents attending the production of each of the Gilbert and Sullivan operas, but mine has been rather an odd career. I have been on the stage over ten years, and have only played regularly nine parts, including the Judge in *Trial by Jury*. At a great benefit *matinée*, I have sometimes taken some small part, but that I count as nothing: but of the above I have, in one or two of the pieces, played the same part night after night, and two performances on Saturday, for a year and a half; while Sir Joseph Porter, in *H.M.S. Pinafore*, I played incessantly for nearly two years.

I have been asked if long runs affect the nerves. I do not think they affect the nerves so much as they affect the performance. Constant repetition begets mechanism, and that is a dreadful enemy to contend against. I try hard to fight against it personally, and believe I succeed. There is one thing I always do— I always play my best to a bad house; for I think it a monstrous thing that an actor should slur through his work because the stalls are empty, and thereby punish those who *have* come for the fault of those who have *not*.

Mrs. Howard Paul impressed so strongly upon me the importance and the justness of playing one's best to a poor house, that I not only have never forgotten her injunction, but have endeavoured to abide by it.

To act without recognition, by applause, laughter, or tears, from an audience is galling to an actor; but, fortunately, I have had a good training in this respect in the private-house engagements, and have got used to it.

In town, my audiences have sometimes displayed a want of enthusiasm, which has been easily understood by everybody but myself; and in my earlier days in the country I used to console myself with the fact that if my entertainments did not *go*, the audience did, which was a comfort and a relief.

I wonder if my friend Frank Thornton will be offended if I repeat an oft-told story about him? I had the pleasure of knowing him in my early entertaining days, and he himself was remarkably clever in short sketches in character.

When I was first engaged at the Opéra Comique to appear in *The Sorcerer*, F. Thornton was "specially retained" to understudy me. I believe he was very nearly engaged himself to play the part. Fortunately for me, he was not.

During the first week he used to come to me each night, and ask how I was. On my replying that I was "all right—never better," it appeared to me that he departed with a disappointed look. His kind enquiries were repeated, as I thought with extra anxiety; but still I kept well, and showed no signs of fatigue. Then he began to insist that I was not looking well; and I replied that, looks or no looks, I felt perfectly well. Finally he came to me with a pill, which he was certain would do for me. I was also certain that it would "*do* for me," and declined to take it; I played nearly two hundred consecutive nights of *The Sorcerer*, and nearly *seven hundred* of *H.M.S. Pinafore*, without missing a single performance.

About the third week of the subsequent piece, *The Pirates of Penzance*, I was called away from the theatre through a domestic affliction; and Frank Thornton, at literally a moment's notice, had to don the Major-General's uniform and play my part. It goes without saying that his was an excellent performance, as those who saw his excessively funny impersonation of the cramped old æsthete in *Patience* will easily understand.

The domestic affliction referred to was the sudden death of my father on April 24th, 1880. At the beginning of this book I stated that I should not deal with the shadows of my life. Nor shall I, beyond stating that the shock to me was so terrible that I often wonder now whether I have quite recovered it. My poor darling mother never did, and she followed him in a year and ten months after.

There was scarcely a paper in Great Britain and Ireland that did not refer to him in the most affectionate terms. If his loss was felt so much by people who knew him only slightly, what must it have been to his two sons, who idolised the very ground he walked upon? His last lecture was on " Dickens and his Works" (Dickens was his favourite subject), and was delivered at Wrexham on April 22nd, two days before his decease; and the kind clergyman who entertained him on the occasion wrote one of the first and sweetest letters of sympathy that I received.

I should like to say that my father was more than astonished at the result of my appearances in *The Sorcerer*, *Pinafore*, and *Pirates*, and was extremely proud of my stage appearances. He was easily pleased, no doubt; but it was a great source of comfort to me to know he *was* pleased.

Soon after the first production of *The Sorcerer* in 1881, I had occasion to go one morning to Maidenhead by train. I occupied a carriage with a lady and three gentlemen, all of one party. The conversation, which I could not help hearing—and unfortunately listeners never hear good of themselves—turned on Gilbert and Sullivan's new and original form of opera. Suddenly, one of the three gentlemen began to criticise my performance in no complimentary terms. The lady, to my joy, differed with my critic, and it appeared for a moment as if all would end happily. Not a bit of it. The two other gentlemen joined in, and began to find fault with my personal appearance as well as my voice (or want of it). The lady still gallantly defended me, but in doing so she only added fuel to the fire; and judging from the tone and manner in which the two last-named gentlemen contradicted her, I could only come to the conclusion that they were her brothers. I suppose I ought to have stopped them; but for the life of me I could not think of a method of doing so. The train, however, began to pull up at Slough; so I determined to change carriages. I took out my card-case, and wrote in pencil on one of my cards, " Thanks awfully," and placed it on the seat beside the two gentlemen previously to making my exit from the compartment. My only regret is, I am not in a position to describe what followed.

This incident reminds me of another, an occasion on which I indirectly denied myself. In 1878, when *H.M.S. Pinafore* was first produced at the Opéra Comique, I always used to give a musical sketch at the piano at the Saturday afternoon performances after the opera. I had some appointment at Kensington, and went to the Temple Station at the conclusion of the performance and got into a first-class carriage of the Underground Railway. Opposite to me sat a middle-aged gentleman with a good-looking lad. The gentleman stared at me hard, and I saw at once that he had recognised me—an easy matter, considering my sketches were, and still are, always given *in propriâ personâ*. He whispered to the boy, and the boy's eyes also became riveted on me. I felt like one of Madame Tussaud's waxworks; although, from the manner in which the gentleman and the boy sat still and stared, they really resembled the effigies more than I did. At last the gentleman moved. He took from his pocket the book of the libretto of *Pinafore* and peered into it, taking good care to hold the outside cover with title towards me, so that I might see what he was reading. Of course, I took not the slightest notice of his actions; but I had great difficulty in restraining a smile as the boy began to whistle the air of " The Ruler of the Queen's Navee." The gentleman was not to be defeated: he handed me the book, and the following conversation took place between the Gentleman and the Clown:

*Gent.:* I beg your pardon; I fancy you must be well acquainted with that play?

*Clown* (turning over leaves of book casually): Oh! yes. I know it very well.

*Gent.:* Well, if *you* do not know it well, I should like to know who does?

*Clown* (handing back book): I do not quite follow you?

*Gent.:* I should have thought you knew it backwards.

*Clown:* That I certainly do not.

*Gent.:* You've heard it often enough?

*Clown:* One cannot help that. It is on all the street bands.

*Gent.:* And seen it too?

*Clown:* No; I am going to see it next Wednesday.

[There was to be a morning performance of one of Mr. D'Oyly Carte's country companies.]

*Gent.:* Well, that's very odd. You'll excuse me, you are exactly like George Grossmith.

*Clown:* I knew you were going to say that. Do you know nearly everybody takes me for Mr. Grossmith?

*Gent.:* I am very sorry. I meant no offence.

*Clown:* Pray don't mention it. I regard it as a great compliment.

*Gent.:* Oh, I'm very glad!

*Railway Porter* (in distance): Sloane Square! Sloane Square!!

*Gent.:* We get out here. Good afternoon.

*Clown:* Good afternoon.

> (*Exeunt* Gentleman and Juvenile by the carriage-door, prompt side. Clown, in spite of the printed warning in front of him, proceeded to place his feet on the opposite cushions.)

A friend of mine, who is (or at all events was) a member of the Scottish Club, mistook Mr. W. S. Penley, the popular actor, for me once on the platform of Waterloo Station. My enthusiastic friend slapped the "Rev. Mr. Spalding" on the back and said:

"Hulloa, Grossmith! How are you? Come and sup after the play next Saturday at Dover Street?"

Penley replied, in the clerical tone characteristic of him:

"I beg your pardon, I'm not Grossmith; but I shall be very pleased to have supper with you."

Another railway recognition story. I was coming up with a party of friends from Ascot, and we were journeying by one of those delightful trains on the S. W. Railway which not only stop at every station, but between each station as well. We stayed at one place a particularly long time; and as a serious-looking station-master faced the window of the carriage in which we were, one of the ladies begged of me to "chaff" him about the slowness of the train. Chaffing is a vulgar habit; but, unfortunately, it is a habit to which I am occasionally addicted. We all have our amusements; and it is not my fault that I do not possess the brave spirit which induces a man to hunt across country and torture a beautiful creature like a deer until, through sheer fright, it takes a leap through the window of a railway station. I prefer to torture one of my own fellow-creatures; for he often stands a fair chance of getting the best of it. The deer never does!

I saw that the serious and stolid station-master was a good subject for chaff; but, as a matter of fact, the whim was not on me. But in deference to the general wish of my friendly travellers, I addressed the station-master as follows:

"I say, station-master, you ought to be ashamed of this line."

The serious official replied:

"So I am."

This scored the first laugh against me. Some of the ladies encouraged me, and said, "Go on, go on;" "Get a rise out of him," &c. I tried again, and this time observed weakly:

"Why don't you get something better to do?"

My victim, never changing his serious aspect, replied:

"You mean, why don't *you* get me something better to do."

This was a real knock-down blow. I came up staggering and a little dazed. My victim, seeing his chance, led the attack:

"Anything more to say?"

I feebly answered:
"No. Have you?"
He said:
"No—except that you act a good deal better here than you do at the Savoy."

The next day I thought of fifty good things I might have said. Alas! how easily things go wrong!

In taking leave of my readers on the subject of my theatrical career, I feel I ought, in justice to myself, to state that all my first appearances are completely marred by uncontrollable nervousness. I am more than nervous—I am absolutely ill.

The first night of *The Mikado* I shall never forget the longest day I live. It must have appeared to all that I was doing my best to spoil the piece. But what with my own want of physical strength, prostration through the numerous and very long rehearsals, my anxiety to satisfy the author, the rows of critics (oh, please do not be hard on me!), rendered *blasé* by the modern custom of half a dozen ridiculous and senseless *matinées* a week, I lose my voice, the little there is of it, my confidence and, what, I maintain, is most valuable of all to me, my own individuality. In fact, I plead guilty to being what Mr. Richard Barker declared me to be on these occasions, "a lamentable spectacle."

In concluding this chapter, let me offer my hearty thanks to Sir Arthur Sullivan for having thought of me, to D'Oyly Carte for having engaged me, to W. S. Gilbert for having advised me, and last, but not least, to the generous public for having tolerated me.

## CHAPTER VII.

### A Society Clown.

> funny fellows, comic men and clowns of private life,
> They 'd none of them be missed—they 'd none of them be missed."
> *The Mikado.*

ONE dull day during the end of the year 1873, the Police Court having adjourned, I went into a ham and beef shop at the corner of Bow Street to get a sandwich. I generally did this when I had not sufficient time to get a proper lunch, so presume I must have been occupied in the very arduous duties of taking notes of an important case, and jotting down suggestions for a new song or sketch at the same moment—at all times a difficult task, involving a deal of confusion. While purchasing my modest meal a little dog entered the shop. Its very tall and slim owner (for he was very slim in those days) whistled to the dog to come out. I presume the dog had reasons for staying in the shop, so the owner had no other option than to walk in and carry the animal out bodily. The owner and I greeted each other:

"How do you do, Mr. Grain?"

"How do you do, Mr. Grossmith?"

We did not know each other so well in those days as we do now, and were naturally a little formal in our method of address.

I enquired, as a matter of course, how his new song was going at the Gallery of Illustration? He enquired how mine was going at the Polytechnic? He then told me that he was busy preparing sketches, for the purpose of giving professionally at private houses during the forthcoming season. I had no idea that this sort of thing was done (I must have been very ignorant, I fear), and in reply to my questions he enlightened me on many points which were of the utmost interest, and subsequent importance to me. I remember asking him if the work was agreeable, and if the people were nice. His answer, I recollect, was very characteristic of him. "Very," he said; "and, what is more important, it pays well." He also told me that John Parry used to sing professionally at private houses. This decided me; for I knew that what was good enough for John Parry and Corney Grain, was more than good enough for me.

"Well," I said, "I think I shall try it, Mr. Grain."

"I certainly should if I were you," he replied.

We said the usual "good-bye at the door;" he departed with his dog into Covent Garden, and I departed with my sandwich into Bow Street.

It so happened that I was going, a few evenings afterwards, to a large musical party near Harley Street, and I decided, if I sang, to try the whole of "The Silver Wedding," the sketch I was then giving at the Polytechnic, instead of the plain comic song which I had generally "obliged with." The hostess, when the time came for me to volunteer, expressed herself much delighted at my proposed innovation. The grand piano was turned as I wanted it, and a little table (supposed to represent the supper table), with wine decanter and glass, was placed to my right. All these preparations, instead of causing the proceedings to flag as one would naturally suppose, only increased the excitement—such as there was, or could be at a private party. I was more than pleased at the result—I was astonished. For instance, I felt sure the imitation after-supper speeches would lose their entire effect from the want of a platform and footlights. The sketch lasted quite half an hour, which I feared would have been thought too long. To my surprise, I was asked if I would mind giving another. However, I let well alone and did not give any more that evening, but took the hint I received from Corney Grain, and began to prepare some sketches specially.

At my next parties I tried "The Puddleton Penny Readings," and "Theatricals at Thespis Lodge," with the same result.

I then went to Mr. George Dolby, who had been Charles Dickens's agent and manager in America, and who had at that time offices in Bond Street, and told him I intended trying the private work. He said it was a capital idea, and he would, in all probability, be able to get me several engagements during the following June and July, which was the busy time for private concerts, &c.

In the meanwhile a clergyman, from Windsor, communicated with me through one of the musical libraries in Bond Street, and secured my services for an evening party at his house; and it is with great satisfaction that I record the circumstance that I was recommended by Corney Grain, who was first applied to, but was unable, for some reason, to accept for himself. After my recent conversation with him on the subject, I thought it most kind of him to perform an action which I should never have dreamed of asking him to do.

The next two seasons I was occupied in forming and increasing a connection. George Dolby sent me several engagements in London, when he found the first one I fulfilled for him passed off without complaint! Then, in time, came the best sign of all that I was progressing; viz., the people began to write to me personally. At first I found it terribly uphill work. If the people do not know the singer they wont listen, on the paradoxical principle that they sometimes wont listen if they *do* know him. Some singers are wonderfully well-known and have a facility for clearing the room almost as remarkable as have some reciters. The "chandelier-shaker" is invariably a "room-clearer." If in my earlier days (or even now for the matter of fact) people displayed no anxiety to hear me, I felt thankful if they did quit the room. Such conduct is preferable to that of the more fashionable people who stop in and talk.

It is a very easy thing for the ordinary drawing-room amateur comic singer to make a success. He has only to watch his opportunity. He will wait, perhaps, till his audience and himself have had supper, and all are in the mood to be amused. But let him go professionally to a dull after-dinner party, where no one knows him, and he finds eight or nine elderly ladies yawning and wondering *when* the gentlemen will come up and join them. Let him try that audience. If he can amuse them, he will not only be satisfied at receiving his cheque, but will be conscious of the fact that he has thoroughly earned it. I feel a special delight in persevering in waking up an audience like that. I resort to all sorts of measures by which I can do so.

Once I was singing at a private house in the country to an odd assortment of people. I was informed that the party followed a wedding which had taken place in the morning. If it had followed a funeral, it would have accounted for the general depression and gloom which prevailed. I played the piano and the fool for three-quarters of an hour, and anything more dismal than the result it would be impossible to imagine. A temptation seized me suddenly, and I said:

"Ladies and Gentlemen,—I am going to reveal to you a secret. Pray don't let it go any further. This is supposed to be a comic entertainment. I don't expect you to laugh at it in the least; but if, during the next sketch, you would only once oblige me with a Society smile, it would give me a great deal of encouragement."

The audience for a moment were dumbfounded. They first began to titter, then to laugh, and actually to roar, and for a time I could not proceed with the sketch. They were transformed into a capital and enthusiastic audience; and the hostess told me that both her guests and herself were most grateful to me.

I am frequently asked if I like giving my entertainments in private houses, and I answer most emphatically that I do. I never feel so much in my element as when I have a nice piano on a dais, and a seated audience of educated and well-dressed people, in a handsome drawing-room. It is a pleasure to me to sing to them; and although I occupy an hour and a half—sometimes more—over the three musical sketches which I usually give, I feel quite sorry when I have finished.

I have never received unkindness from anyone—quite the reverse. So much hospitality and good-will have been extended towards me by people who are utter strangers, and whose associations with me have been purely of a business character, that I often have wondered what I have done to deserve it all.

There are the usual "four to seven" afternoon parties. I have a little dread of what is known as the "smart" evening parties in London. The large suites of rooms will be comparatively empty at eleven o'clock; but in a quarter of an hour the guests will stream in in hundreds. Then they block up all the rooms and staircases, while thirty or forty will crowd round the grand piano and exclude the rest from any chance of seeing or hearing the unfortunate singer. In half or three-quarters of an hour the rooms will be empty again. But I must say a "smart" party is at all times an interesting sight: the beautiful dresses, the array of diamonds, the stars and garters, especially if a Royal function is taking place the same evening, so that people are "going on" or "have come on from." Yet with all this grandeur it does seem such an anomaly, among so much greatness, so much wealth, to hear such a babel of idiotic conversation even from the mouths of the most able representatives of the Houses of Lords and Commons. The greater the people, the smaller the talk.

Music on such an occasion is quite out of place, and I never can understand why the hostess arranges to have any. A grand reception, I take it, is a reception, and not a concert. It is impossible to combine the two. I do not blame the people on these occasions for talking: they cannot even get into the room where the music is. Sometimes, by adopting the fashionable process of spitefully digging your way through people, you may get near the piano, and even a glimpse of the singer. Yes, there he is—a well-known drawing-room tenor, perhaps, who has received fifty guineas to sing a couple of songs. You see him simply indulging, apparently, in a dumb-show performance. The windows are open behind him, and there is a perfect din of the "clinking" of the harness of hundreds of horses in the road outside, intermingled with lusty shouts from the linkmen, with trombone voices, far and near: "Lady Peckham Rye's carriage next;" "Col. Waterloo Rhodes's carriage stops the way;" "Mrs. Bompleton's servant," "Coming out," "Coming in," "Baron Bosch's carriage —no servant."

Fortunately I cannot arrive at such parties until about a quarter to twelve at night (having, of course, my usual engagement at the Savoy to fulfil), and by that time the rooms have cleared a little, either through departure of guests for another party or for supper below. The chairs are suddenly produced in a semi-circle round the piano, and I am turned on to wind up the evening, having previously wound up myself. And I do wind up myself sometimes, even to the extent of getting the livelier and more juvenile members of the aristocracy, as the end of my entertainment approaches, to join, without invitation, in the chorus of "The Duke of Seven Dials," "See me Dance the Polka," or "The Happy Fatherland," according to the jingling nature of the song.

It was at a reception of this sort at a ducal mansion that I overheard a rather rude enquiry respecting myself. I arrived after my performance at the theatre, and I was leaving the drawing-room with her Grace in order to arrange for a slight alteration of the position of the piano, which had been placed so that only the back of my head could be seen, and I am willing to confess that I have not much expression there. The Duke, who is tolerably well-known for his brusque and autocratic manner, addressing her Grace in my presence, said, " Has that fellow arrived yet ? " The Duchess looked terribly confused, and glanced at the Duke and myself alternately, but I did not answer. As the Duke repeated the question with the amount of severity that a husband is always privileged to use towards his wife, I replied politely, " Yes, your Grace, that fellow has arrived." With that I walked away and directed the servants to move the piano, and out of revenge I determined to exert my utmost to make my entertainment go well. Although his Grace was rude to his wife, of course he did not intend to be rude to me; for immediately the first sketch was over he came and told me how pleased he was with it.

Although I have never been treated with any rudeness, still I have been often amused by the peculiarities of people.

A gentleman wrote to me for the purpose of engaging me, and, rightly or wrongly, asked me if my sketches were quite *comme il faut*, as he had several young daughters. I was so immensely tickled by this, that, also rightly or wrongly, I replied that my entertainments *were* as they should be; for I was recently married, and hoped myself to have several young daughters. He wrote thanking me for this assurance, and I was to consider myself accordingly engaged.

I never like arriving early at these afternoon engagements; and if I arrive late, my hostess gets naturally anxious. It depresses me to have to stand in a drawing-room which has been cleared of every stick of furniture for the occasion, and to watch the arrival of the solemn-looking ladies and their daughters, who generally attend such gatherings early. The young men never turn up till about five or half-past. In order to avoid this, I write to my hostess to tell her of the time I shall arrive, which I fix at about half or three quarters of an hour after the hour for which her invitations have been issued. The consequence is that when I arrive the room is full; people have warmed themselves into a general conversation, and I walk straight to the piano and commence my first half-hour without more ado.

Sometimes—very rarely—a lady will politely request me to arrive a little before the time: of course I comply with this request, and make the best of it, but during the latter part of June and the first few weeks in July it is no joke. I have arrived punctually at a "four to seven" party, and have not commenced my first sketch till a quarter to six; the day having been fine and the guests all driving in the park. During those months people do not arrive until five, and then they appear to have one eye on me and the other on the tea. The audience is composed almost entirely of ladies—but I like them.

Some years ago I was most particularly requested by one anxious and evidently very nervous lady to arrive punctually on a certain afternoon. I arrived, and was received most cordially by the hostess, who, to my delight, had the room arranged with chairs so that the people could sit down; but on my arrival only one chair was occupied, and that was by a boy in an Eton jacket, who was seated by himself at the extreme end of the room. I waited full three-quarters of an hour before a single person arrived. In the meanwhile the lady handed me a little pink envelope enclosing what Sir Digby Grant, in *The Two Roses*, designates "a little cheque." I placed it hastily in my pocket, and was much amused by the lady approaching me shortly afterwards and saying, "Have you got it quite safe?"

I enquired what?

She replied, " The little envelope."

I said, " Oh yes, thank you."

" Oh, that is all right," she said. " It seemed to me you placed it rather carelessly in your pocket."

" Oh, it was not carelessness," I assured her; " only bashfulness."

At a quarter to five two ladies arrived, and at five the hostess, addressing me, said:

" Would you mind commencing now? Some of the audience have been here nearly an hour."

This, I presume, had reference to the Eton boy at the back of the room, who came before time.

" With pleasure," I remarked. I opened the grand piano and commenced the first item. I had not been at it more than ten minutes when the two ladies got up, and, shaking hands with the hostess, said they were so sorry they could not stay any longer, but they had to meet some friends at another party before half-past five. I therefore continued the next twenty minutes of the sketch to the solitary boy, whose totally immovable face gave me no idea as to whether he was enjoying the entertainment or not. The room soon began to fill with extraordinary rapidity. At the conclusion of the entertainment the hostess again, in a whisper, asked if I still had the envelope quite safe. I pulled it half-way out of my breast coat-pocket, and said, with a smile and a nod, " It's all right, you see."

She laughed and replied:

" Oh, yes; I see it's all right."

At the foot of the stairs I encountered the Eton boy with the serious face. He had stayed till the very last. I said:

"Well, weren't you bored with all the rot I've been talking?"

He replied:

"No; it was awfully jolly. I wish there had been more of it."

There was no affectation about the boy, and his simple answer gave me much satisfaction.

If I had not spoken, he would have said nothing. How very different from the lady who has been talking on the staircase at the top of her voice, who has never once listened or even glanced towards the piano, but who, on seeing you pass by, greets you with:

"What a wonderful man you are! How *can* you think of all these things? You are quite too delightful!"

I have frequently been amused at the amount of diffidence displayed by people when handing me the honorarium. Sometimes the hostess will thank me profusely, and, in shaking hands, squeeze the little envelope into my palm.

Some ladies will say loudly, "Good-bye, and thank you so much." Then softly, "I will write you to-morrow."

Some ladies will whisper mysteriously, "You will hear from my husband to-morrow." This at first sounds rather awful; but the husband's communication is pleasant and most welcome.

The *Pall Mall Gazette* published a most amusing sketch of an elderly gentleman paying me in specie in the middle of the room, and dropping the sovereigns all over the floor.

A very wealthy gentleman drove up to my father's house, about fifteen years ago, in a carriage and pair and with gorgeous livery, for the purpose of securing my services. I was out of town at the time; so my father mentioned my fee, which was not very exorbitant in those days. The gentleman was not inclined to give more than half; so my discriminating parent "closed" with him. I do not mean in the pugilistic sense of the word, but that he accepted the terms on my behalf. I fulfilled the engagement; and when I saw the lovely mansion, with its magnificent drawing-room, I wondered a little at my host having suggested a reduction in the fee. I do not wonder now: I have experienced still more wonderful things since then. The gentleman himself was very kind, as far as I remember. I was only a beginner, and in all probability he did not even know my name perfectly. He paid me on the first landing, and a shilling slipped through his fingers and rolled down the staircase. I was about to roll down after it, when he stopped me, saying:

"Please don't trouble; here's another."

As I went out of the door I beheld my host and about four liveried servants hunting for the lost coin.

As far as my own feelings are concerned, I experience no particular delicacy as to the manner in which I am paid. I prefer the cheque to be sent on a day or two after; and I least like the medical-man custom of slipping the fee into the hand as you depart. You cannot, under such circumstances, shake hands naturally or with comfort; and there is always the chance of a sovereign falling on the oilcloth, to say nothing of the risk of banging your heads together as you both politely dive after it. Why should I be bashful, when I see members of the aristocracy selling goods over a counter, and taking the money and giving change in exactly the same manner as the ordinary tradesman?

A young gentleman once called upon me. He explained that he was acting as a sort of ambassador for a friend of his, Mrs. ——, of Mayfair, who wished me to dine at her house. I replied that I had not the honour of the lady's acquaintance, and, though appreciating her kind invitation, did not exactly see how I could very well avail myself of it. He said that Prince Somebody-orother and La Comtesse de Soandso would be dining there, and Mrs. —— would be so pleased if I would join the party, and sing a little song after dinner.

"Oh," I said, "if Mrs. —— wishes to engage me professionally, that is another matter, and, if I am at liberty, I will come with much pleasure."

"Oh," said the ambassador, "I fancy Mrs. —— is under the impression that if she includes you in her dinner-party, it is an understood thing that you sing afterwards."

"I am afraid I do not understand that," I said. "It would not pay me to do so. I only consume about ten shillings' worth of food and wine, and my terms are more than that."

Sometimes, at private houses, I am retained to take part in a concert, and not give the entire entertainment myself; and it is astonishing to what expense a hostess will sometimes go to entertain and amuse her guests.

I used to be engaged every year by a lady who lived in quite a small house, in a street turning out of Lowndes Square. Beyond a choice collection of old china, there was no outward display of wealth. Her guests at her afternoon parties I should not imagine exceeded forty in number, and these were always made to sit down. She declared she would not have her entertainments spoiled by a crowd, and she was perfectly right.

One afternoon when I was singing there she had a well-known soprano, tenor and pianist, a lady and gentleman who gave recitals in costume, and Señor Sarasate, the violinist. On another occasion she engaged several well-known singers, also Madame Norman Neruda (who, I remember, played exquisitely on that occasion), while the comic element was supplied by Miss Fanny Leslie and myself. On neither of the above afternoons could the entertainment have cost the hostess much less than £150.

Sometimes I am engaged with only one singer, who, the host will explain, will be able to effectually fill up my intervals of rest. Clifford Harrison (the most talented and most popular of drawing-room reciters) and I, have been engaged together—a combination which has been most agreeable to me. I have also been engaged on two or three occasions with Corney Grain, which was a case (as he humorously put it) of " one down, the other come on."

Once I received a letter saying, " Besides yourself, I have secured an *ocarina*."

I do not know if I have spelt it properly, but, for the life of me, I could not tell what an ocarina was. I found it was an oval-shaped instrument, of jet black, which emitted sounds like the notes of a flute with a very bad cold. The performer looked, while playing it, as if he were eating a large potato.

Perhaps the most interesting professional engagement I have ever fulfilled in private was at the residence of Mr. John Aird, M.P., Hyde Park Terrace, on the 17th June, 1887. It was Jubilee year, and the amiable and generous host was evidently determined to treat his guests to a novel entertainment. He wanted something that had not been done before, and instructed his friend, Rutland Barrington, to look out for an original entertainment. A suggestion came eventually from Mr. Fred. Leslie, the clever actor, that the screen scene from *The School for Scandal* should be performed in dumb show. Barrington and Leslie discussed the matter, and it was arranged that there should be no costumes, and that the silent actions of the performers should be described by a lecturer. Mr. Aird was delighted with the idea, and determined that the piece should be well cast. I feel sure the reader will be interested to know who took part in the performance; so I append the cast:

| | |
|---|---|
| Sir Peter Teazle ... ... | Mr. ARTHUR CECIL. |
| Joseph Surface ... ... ... | Mr. FRED. LESLIE. |
| Charles Surface ... ... | Mr. CORNEY GRAIN. |
| Servant ... ... ... ... | Mr. DURWARD LELY. |
| Lady Teazle ... ... ... | Mr. GEORGE GROSSMITH. |
| Lecturer ... ... ... ... | Mr. RUTLAND BARRINGTON. |
| At the Piano ... | Mr. MUNROE COWARD. |

The skit had been carefully rehearsed several times, and Mr. Aird ("our manager," as we called him) attended all the rehearsals in the most business-like manner, and gave some valuable suggestions. The performance, which lasted about twenty-five minutes, went with a roar of laughter from beginning to end.

I thought it stood a chance of being successful, but had no idea it would succeed so well as it did. Barrington's introduction and description were very funny. He commenced by explaining that a dramatic license had at the last moment been refused us, and we were not, therefore, permitted to speak any dialogue; but he would stand at the side and explain the plot and performance as they proceeded. He also added that another disappointment had been experienced by the non-arrival of the costumes, and apologised for the screen being a glass one, but it was the only one he could get. Although our actions were at times extravagant, still we played with great seriousness. There was no ridiculous "mugging," which always spoils a burlesque performance. There was no conventional comic walk, strut, or pantaloon gait. We discarded the usual knowing grin which always seems to say, "I'm the funny man; prepare to laugh." An audience never requires to be told in this fashion that a man is funny; they are quite capable of discovering the fact for themselves. A carroty wig and a red nose can no more make a comedian than a coat can make a man. It was the extreme seriousness of the opening scene between Leslie and Cecil, as Joseph and Sir Peter, that set the audience off at the very beginning. Fred. Leslie was simply immense. His natural look of extreme horror when Sir Peter indicated he suspected Charles

Surface simply convulsed the people. Arthur Cecil was excessively funny in his relation of his quarrels with her ladyship. He was as melancholy as all the Sir Peters ever played put together; and the following was the climax:

*The Lecturer* (Barrington): Sir Peter will now express that in their last quarrel, Lady Teazle almost hinted that she should not break her heart if he was dead.

Arthur Cecil did a little dumb-show action, then quietly rose from his chair and lay at full length on the stage, on his back.

When the servant entered, and Charles Surface was announced, Barrington said:

"Joseph Surface says, ''Sdeath, blockhead! I'm not within.'" [Suitable action by Leslie.]

*Lecturer:* Joseph Surface says he is "out for the day." Observe, ladies and gentlemen, how Joseph describes being out for the day.

Here Leslie put on his opera-hat, seized an imaginary partner, and began waltzing round, *à la* Rosherville Gardens.

Charles Surface was eventually introduced.

*Lecturer:* Charles Surface now enters. Please observe, ladies and gentlemen, that Charles Surface is "fast."

The entrance of Corney Grain, with his hat very much on one side, and his thumbs stuck in his waistcoat, as emblems of fastness, may be imagined better than described. In fact, it is quite impossible to describe the performance. All I can say is, that it had to be repeated; and, whether it was artistic or not, Mr. Luke Fildes, R.A., and Mr. Marcus Stone, R.A., attended **both performances.**

It may be asked how we managed to conclude the performance.  After the screen was thrown down—for which, of course, there was no necessity; for through the glass could distinctly be seen her ladyship, with a plate of sandwiches and a glass of wine—the Lecturer said :

"All having been satisfactorily explained——"

At this abrupt announcement, without any action to justify it, there was continued laughter.

"According to the present fashion which prevails in revivals of old comedies, a minuet *à la mode* will be danced."

Munroe Coward arranged "Oh, the Jubilee!" a seasonable and popular comic song, *à la* minuet, in a most skilful manner; and to this we danced and made our bows, with the exception of myself, who, arrayed in an antimacassar, indulged in my very best *courtesy*.

Our host and hostess, whose reputation for kindness and hospitality cannot be surpassed, placed everything in our way to help us, and were so interested themselves that I know I can say, on the part of the players, that our labour was one of love.  Our audience showed pretty plainly that they enjoyed the performance, and I know we did.

I have given entertainments at the houses of all sorts and conditions of men, and all sorts of places.  Once I sang at a large christening party.  I should think sixty or seventy people sat down to lunch.  The health of the baby was, of course, proposed, and the baby was produced and handed round to all the guests to kiss.  It stood this trying ordeal with perfect good humour; but the darling little boy was obliged to draw the line somewhere, and so he drew it at me. He set up a series of howls which alarmed the whole party—especially the nurse, who darted at me a look of unmistakable indignation. If I had surreptitiously pinched the little treasure, the look of the nurse could not have been more terrible. She departed with the baby, and soothed it with the following pleasant remark about myself:

"Was 'im frightened by an ugly man den?"

I am very fond of children, and I flatter myself that children are fond of me, as a rule. But there are exceptions, of course; and I will relate another of them.

A great friend of mine, whose country house is not a thousand miles away from Twyford, has a bonny little boy, who, at the age of about a year and a half, took a sudden dislike to my *pince nez*, and began to squall the moment I entered the room. From a humorous spirit of mischief, the fond mother in future held me up as a bogey to the boy. If he was fractious, the following threat was held out to him:

"If you are not good, *I will call Mr. Grossmith;*" or, "If you do not eat your food, I shall send you into the room where *Mr. Grossmith is.*"

This always had the desired effect. I believe I have been useful in various ways, but this is the only time I have been required as a bogey to frighten children. As a sequel to the story, I may say the boy is a little older now, and we are very good friends; in fact, the last time I saw him he, of his own accord, selected me as his companion to spend an entire afternoon in the garden collecting snails.

An amusing series of incidents was the result of an engagement which I fulfilled at the residence of a gentleman in Kent. On going to the Opéra Comique one evening, I found a gentleman waiting for me at the stage-door. He introduced himself as the head clerk of Mr. A——, a distinguished manufacturer, who was desirous of obtaining my services for an evening party, to be given in honour of the coming of age of young Mr. A——, at the family mansion in Kent. I invited the head clerk to my dressing-room; for, as we were about to close the theatre for a short time, I knew there was a possibility of my being able to accept the engagement. The clerk at once commenced the conversation by saying that he did a little acting himself—" only as an amateur, of course." I had no reason to doubt his statement, seeing that he had shaved his moustache off and grown his hair to an inordinate length behind.

"Now," said he, coming to the business point of the transaction, "Mr. A—— wants to know how much you charge, first."

I enlightened him on that matter.

"Well, I dare say that'll be all right. Mr. A—— means to spare no expense. But the great thing is—what sort of entertainment do you give?"

I explained that I took my seat at the piano, and chatted, played, and sang, after the manner of John Parry.

"Is there no change of costumes? Don't you require any scenery or footlights?"

"No," I replied. "I'm simply like one of the guests, except that I do something and they don't."

"Oh," said the clerk, a little puzzled, "one of the guests? I must see Mr. A—— about that. I don't think he understands that."

"Well," I observed, "you had better see that he understands that before we proceed any further."

The head clerk said, "Good-night," and left the room, with a gait that seemed to hit the happy medium between the walk of Henry Irving and the stride of a pantomimic policeman.

The next night he returned, with profuse apologies, stating that Mr. A—— of course would receive me as a guest, and would feel honoured at making my acquaintance.

This was rather going to extremes, I thought; but the fault was on the right side. I booked the date, and eventually "attended the evening party." I shall never forget it. I was received as a guest—as *the* guest, in fact—and no mistake about it. My reception was enormous. Young Mr. A——, who had come of age, was, comparatively speaking, nowhere. I was introduced to nearly everybody—or, more strictly speaking, nearly everybody was *presented* to me. My entertainments were never better received. They were given at intervals during the dancing. I danced with the most attractive dancers, whom the host compelled to dance with me.

I enjoyed it immensely.

I don't think they did, and am positive their displaced partners did not.

Shortly after midnight the supper-rooms were thrown open, and I was requested to take the hostess in to supper. No royal prince could have been treated better than I was. An elderly clergyman quoted from my entertainment in proposing the health of young Mr. A——, on the auspicious occasion of his coming of age. Young Mr. A—— followed the clergyman's example in returning thanks. Then, to my utter surprise, Mr. A—— sen., proposed my health, and thanked me for coming down.

I returned thanks; and as there was a risk of an anti-climax, I rose—with an amount of consummate impudence which, I am sorry to say, is a little characteristic of me—and proposed the health of the host and hostess, on the plea that I was the oldest friend of the family, and had known them all their lives. This observation was received with continued roars of laughter. I did not, and do not even now, think it funny; but please remember, after a good champagne supper, people will roar at anything.

We returned to the drawing-room. I sang again, and then came the hour for my departure, for I had to drive all the way to town.

Mr. A—— stood in the middle of the room and shouted:

"Silence for a moment. All those who have been delighted with Mr. Grossmith, please hold up their hands."

Up went all the hands with the exception of those belonging to the displaced partners. Mr. A——, with much forethought, for which I mentally thanked him, refrained from appealing to the "noes."

Continuing his thanks, Mr. A—— said:

"We are all much obliged to you, Mr. Grossmith; and"—here he fumbled in his right-hand pocket—"and if ever you want a little rest, we shall give you a hearty welcome if you like to stay here; and"—here he seized my right hand, and I felt an envelope being forced into it—"and mind you come. Good-bye. I think you'll find that right," referring to the cheque, of course.

On eventually examining the cheque, I found it was written for an amount nearly double my fee.

I daresay many will think the cordiality extended towards me by Mr. A—— was ostentatious, if not absolutely vulgar. All I can say is, it was infinitely to be preferred to the reception I once received from a lady of title who invited me to her party, who had not engaged me professionally, but who welcomed me at the top of the staircase with a vacant look and the following observation in her most aristocratic tone:

"How late you are! Will you sing now?"

I need scarcely say there was no song; but there was a supper, of which I took full advantage.

Yet another incident, which occurred in my dressing-room at the Opéra Comique, and which is indelible on my memory:

A laird sent his Scotch butler to me one evening to make inquiries respecting my entertainment. The butler, an elderly, pompous, and exceedingly stupid man, produced a piece of note-paper containing a string of questions which he was instructed to ask me.

The first question was: "Can Mr. Grossmith give an entertainment at Aberdeen on Jan.——?"

I replied that my nightly engagement at the theatre would totally prevent my accepting an engagement at Aberdeen. I could only sing at afternoon parties in town, or a short distance from it.

The butler, with a broad Scotch accent, which I need not imitate here, said:

"Ye'll have the goodness to answer this question, please. 'Can Mr. Grossmith give an entertainment at Aberdeen on Jan. ——?'"

"No; I cannot," I replied.

The butler continued reading:

"'What will be his terms?'"

"But I cannot go," I argued.

"Ye'll save a deal o' time if ye'll answer the questions, please. What'll be the terms?"

"Well, we will say a hundred guineas, as I can't go," I answered, endeavouring to restrain myself from bursting out laughing in his face.

The butler made a note of the terms, and continued:

"'Will the entertainment be consistent?'"

"What?" I ejaculated.

"'Will the entertainment be consistent?'"

"Consistent?" For the life of me, I could not see what he meant.

"Yes—consistent."

I thought a little, and then said:

"Would you kindly explain the question? I do not understand it in the least."

The butler said:

"Well, you must know, the laird is a strict Presbyterian, and all the guests will be strict

Presbyterians, and he wants to know if your entertainment will be consistent."

"Now I understand you," I replied. "Certainly, my entertainment will be quite consistent. I am always very careful, and shall only sing *Presbyterian comic songs*."

He made a note of my remark in the most serious way, and left, saying:

"The laird himself will write to say if he can accept the terms."

That occurred nearly ten years ago, and the laird has not written yet.

Giving entertainments in private houses is a constant source of delight to me, and I feel both pleasure and pride in my work. I take sometimes enormous pains in writing and composing the sketches, and have often devoted several hours a day for a week or so in arranging and composing a musical illustration which will only occupy a few minutes in performance, and which may pass almost unnoticed by the majority of the audience. But when the connoisseur picks that illustration out from all the rest of the entertainment as his choice, I feel I am more than rewarded for my trouble.

All sorts of stories about me appear from time to time in the cheap weekly journals of the coloured paper or wrapper type, and I suppose they are amusing to the readers. They amuse *me* sometimes. I never mind chaff.

My entertainments in private are capital scope for the smaller journalists; and journalists, like other people, can be very small sometimes. I read accounts of my own indignation at having been told to go round to the servants' entrance; how a duchess was horrified at discovering she was dancing with me instead of Lord Adolphus; my injured feelings because a hostess did not shake hands with me; and my having called upon the butler at Marlborough House, and spreading the report that I had visited the Prince of Wales. These paragraphs, though absolutely untrue, are inoffensive, and do good, inasmuch as they do not hurt me, but supply the author with a few hard and honestly-earned shillings.

Spiteful and really offensive paragraphs are regarded by me in a different light. An offensive paragraph has the same effect upon me as an anonymous letter. I feel the same sort of pity for the writer as I do for the poor "Norfolk Howard," who can only do its work in the dark, and cuts such a terrified figure when the light is suddenly flashed upon it. The anonymous letter-writer is, perhaps, the worst of the three; for his action is nearly always dictated by a feeling of spite; whereas the "Norfolk Howard" and the "offensive paragraphist" are actuated by a feeling of hunger: and *necessitas non habet leges*.

There are exceptions to every rule, and I soon ascertained that hunger was not the *raison d'être* of the following exceptional notice in reference to my *début* in a weekly paper:

" *      *      *      *      *      *      *

\*   \*   \*   And something which was called an 'entertainment' by a beardless boy, whose tones betokened his Cockney birth, and whose sole ideas of humour seemed to be derived from an excessive abuse of vulgar gesture, and the constant employment of such slang terms as are heard in police-courts and penny gaffs. When Master Grossmith was not vulgar, he was simply stupid; for which reason his attempts at amusing an intelligent audience by a wretched imitation of the Christy Minstrels and a badly-arranged rehash of Albert Smith's 'Evening Parties' were, as they deserved to be, a dead failure. The whole exhibition was most painful, and as far beneath what we should have expected to see at the Polytechnic as a 'Penny Dreadful' is from one of Thackeray's novels. Our advice to the *debutant* is, to tarry at Jericho till his beard be grown."

I was extremely hurt at this, but the direct allusion to the police-court aroused my suspicions. I became a sort of amateur detective; and the result was, I "received information" that the article had been written by a gentleman of position, who had just beforehand been charged at Bow Street with a very serious offence, and whose friends had not been successful in persuading me to "keep the case out of the paper," or in "altering his name" beyond recognition.

I owe very much to the Press, not merely for the favour extended towards me, but also for improvements gathered from their adverse criticism. But whenever I read a notice like the above, I am consoled by the thought that its author, at some time or other, without consent or consultation, has put in an appearance at Bow Street Police Court during my reign as reporter.

In the foregoing chapter, I have dealt entirely

with visits into Society professionally. In the next, and last, I shall speak of the non-professional invitations: for, strange as it may appear to the uninitiated, I am *not* always expected "to oblige with a song;" nor is it a *sine quâ non* that if I accept an invitation to dinner, it is on the distinct understanding that I should be funny. I can be a very rational being when I choose; and any hostess who asked me to her residence in the expectation that I should gratuitously amuse her guests, would find me particularly prosaic.

Happily for all professional men and women, such hostesses are very rare; and, fortunately, their reputations precede them. Still, there *are* people who cannot understand why I should appear *in propriâ personâ* in a drawing-room; and a wealthy hatter of slight acquaintance, meeting me at a "Mansion House" ball, said:

"Hulloa! Mr. Grossmith, what are *you* doing here? Are you going to give us any of your little funniments—eh?"

"No," I replied. "Are you going to sell any of your hats?"

## CHAPTER VIII.

### A Very Snobbish Chapter.

*"I've got a little list."—The Mikado.*

CAPTAIN HAWLEY SMART, at the Garrick one day, at lunch, gave me a valuable friendly warning.

"In your book," said he, "do not fall into that diary mistake, characteristic of most autobiographers; and some autobiographers indulge in it very badly. I mean writing: 'May 14th.—Dined at the Duke of A——'s: present, Lord and Lady B——, Count C——, Marquis of D——, &c.' Much better write down a list of all the people you *have* met, and say: 'Dined with, or met, this lot some time or other.'"

Unfortunately, I do not keep a diary, and have no list of "people I have known;" but I can truthfully say that during the last twelve or fourteen years I have had the privilege of meeting what the Society papers repeatedly call "everybody, who is anybody." What! everybody? Well, nearly everybody! I have met Royal Princes in their palaces, and Republicans in their republic houses. I am personally acquainted with Bishops and Bradlaugh. I have shaken hands with Sarah Bernhardt and Miss Bessie Bellwood. I have been visited by millionaires who are nobodies, and by beggars who are somebodies. I have exchanged courtesies with Gustave Doré, and another celebrated painter has exchanged umbrellas with me. I know Sims Reeves and "Squash." I manage to get on with peers and peasants; I talk a little about the weather to the former, and a little (very little) about the crops to the latter.

I believe I am a Conservative, but I own to a great admiration for Gladstone. I am not alone in that respect, except that I "own up" my admiration, and other Conservatives do not. I regret exceedingly that I never met Lord Beaconsfield; but when I commenced to "go out," he had almost ceased doing so. I met Mr. Gladstone at a garden party as recently as the autumn of 1887, and was asked to meet him in June, 1888. It is a pleasure to converse with him, or, rather, to hear him converse with you. At the former party, a lady said to me, "If that horrid man comes here, I shall walk through that window on to the lawn. I would not stay under the same roof with him." She evidently thought there was no chance of his coming; in point of fact, she afterwards admitted as much to me. When he *did* arrive, she followed him about, curtsied as he passed, as if he were the Queen, repeatedly offered him her chair, and indulged in that particular kind of adoration in the *presence* which is usually indulged in by people who are ultra-bitter during the *absence*.

But though I have not kept a list of the notable people I have met, I have kept the letters of those who have written to me as a friend or acquaintance. I cannot count myself as one of the "pestilential nuisances who apply for autographs," as Gilbert describes them in *The Mikado;* still, I must plead guilty to pasting in a book, or keeping in my desk, every letter addressed to me personally that has a good name attached. When I say every letter, I do not include letters addressed to me professionally or purely on business matters: those are of merely passing value to me. I simply treasure the letters of those with whom I have become actually acquainted. This collection is the collection of a Snob, no doubt; and I can only beg of those of my readers who are sensitive to Snobbish actions to pass this chapter over, for my sake as well as theirs.

I would add that my wife and I do not possess a card-basket, where the only countess's card will keep shifting up to the top, of its own accord, in the most remarkable fashion; nor do we advertise our evening parties in the *Morning Post*, nor publicly announce that we have removed to a hired cottage at Datchet during the fixture of a telephone pole to the roof of our family mansion in Dorset (pronounced Dossit) Square.

I will take the letters as they come, simply calling attention to the contents or the writers as I imagine they may interest or amuse the readers. The first—the most interesting to me, perhaps, as it turned the tide of my professional life—is the letter from Arthur Sullivan, asking me to go on the stage, which has already appeared in a former chapter. The next is from J. R. Planché, whom I shall always remember with the greatest pleasure, and whose little parties were delightful.

The following is characteristic of J. R. Planché's well-known courtesy:

6 Royal Avenue,<br>
Chelsea, S.W.,<br>
*5th August,* 1875.

Dear Mr. Grossmith,—Nothing could give me more pleasure than doing anything which is agreeable to you. I estimate highly your talent, and am flattered by your friendship. With kindest regards from all of us to you and your amiable and gifted wife,
Believe me,<br>
Very sincerely yours,<br>
J. R. Planché.

---

The above is very flattering, and so is the following from Frederic Clay; and if I were a truly modest man, I should publish neither:

64 Seymour Street,<br>
Portman Square.

Dear Grossmith,—Miss Kate Santley has asked me to write her a light song for the piece she is now playing. Since Miss Santley immortalised "Nobody knows as I know" for me, my humble pen has always been at her disposal—in fact, I have composed a couple of operas for her—but just now I am night and day at work on this Brighton Cantata; nor can I dream where to find words without being vulgar.

As you were good enough to give me more real amusement and enjoyment at Arthur Blunt's than I have known for many a long day, I could not help suggesting your name to Miss Santley, telling her that, if you can find time for the purpose, she could not be in safer or more accomplished hands than yours. . . .

Yours very sincerely,<br>FREDERIC CLAY.

I afterwards became very intimate with Frederic Clay; and a great portion of one of his subsequent works (the *Black Crook*, I think) was composed while he was staying with my wife and myself at a tiny cottage which we rented during the autumn each year at Datchet. His last work of all he chiefly did at Datchet. It was called, I think, *The Golden Ring*, and the book was by G. R. Sims. He hired a cottage a few doors from mine, and as I passed to and fro of a morning I used to see him writing hard at his desk in front of the open window, and invariably greeted him with "Good-morning, Freddy; do you want any of your harmonies corrected?"—"Shall I score the drum parts for you?"—or some such nonsense. It will be remembered that he was seized with a serious illness after the production of the piece at the Alhambra. I grieve to say I seldom see him now, as he lives away in the country very quietly. He wrote a charming letter in pencil some months ago respecting a favourable notice he had seen of the pianoforte-playing of my little girl Sylvia at a "pupils'" concert. I have kept many of his letters, and value them. I wanted to see him about something, and suggested we should meet at the Beefsteak Club. This was his reply:

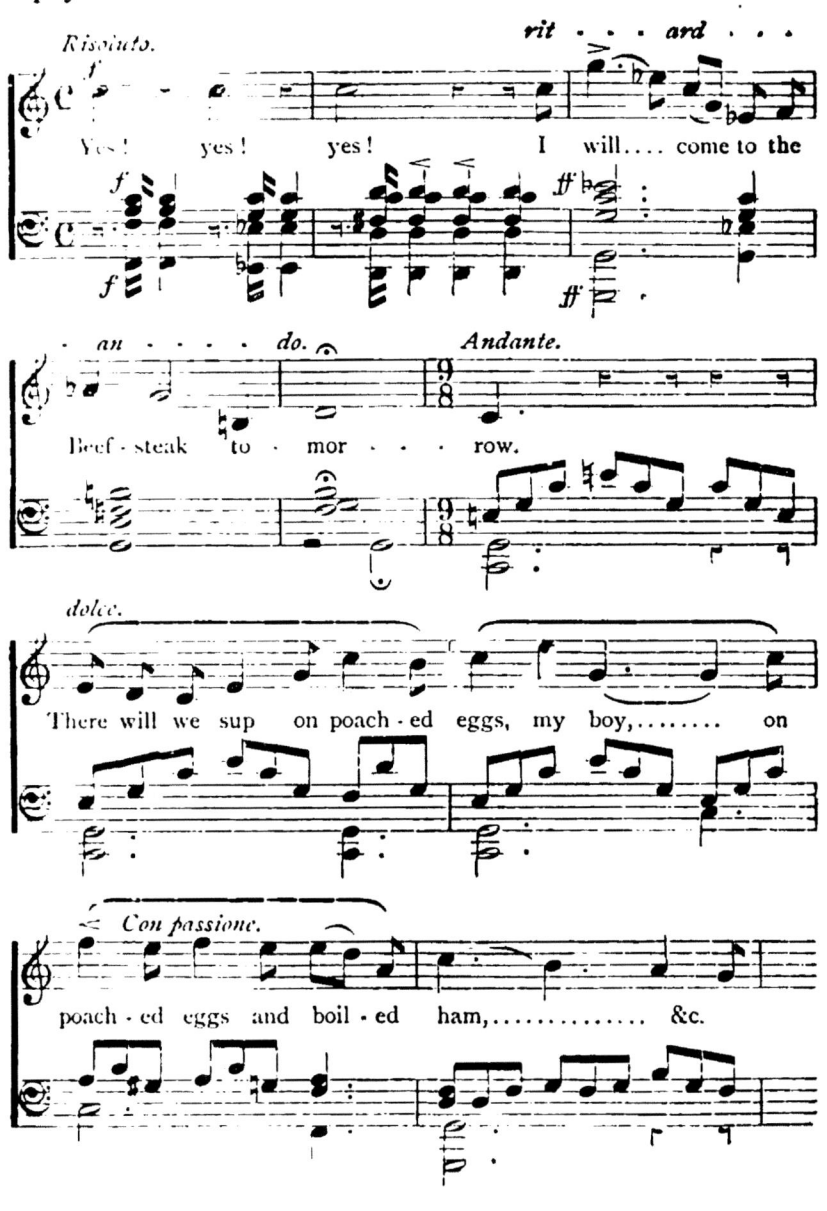

*[musical score with lyrics: "Yes! yes! yes! I will.... come to the Beef-steak to-mor-row. There will we sup on poach-ed eggs, my boy, ........ on poach-ed eggs and boil-ed ham, ............. &c."]*

At the old Gallery of Illustration, in 1875, Corney Grain was suddenly indisposed, and I sang for him; and I was very pleased at the thought of giving a sketch at the very piano on which John Parry had played. Subsequently I received the following letter from Mrs. German Reed:

. . . Please accept my best thanks, and with them a handkerchief which Mr. John Parry used in his song, "Mrs. Roseleaf's Evening Party." You said you would be pleased to have it. The little piece of cotton in the middle he always had tied to prevent confusion in folding while singing.
With kind compliments to your wife,
Sincerely yours,
PRISCILLA REED.

---

I sang and acted at the Gallery of Illustrations on another occasion. Corney Grain was required to give his "Sketches at a Country House," where he was to meet the Prince of Wales; and I undertook, besides giving my sketch "Theatricals at Thespis Lodge," to act the part of the young lover (Grain's part) in *Very Catching*, an excellent little piece by F. C. Burnand, and music by Molloy. In this, both Mrs. German Reed and Arthur Cecil played. I had to sing a sentimental duet with Miss Fanny Holland, "O'er the stones go tripping," during which she had to rest on my shoulder as I led her from stone to stone. But there happened to be a great difference in the height of Grain and myself; and when Miss Holland found that she could not stoop low enough to reach my shoulders, and that the strip of artificial water, which was arranged to well cover Grain's ankles, was up to my knees, she fairly burst out laughing on the stage.

Next come rather amusing letters from the late Duchess of Westminster and Lady Diana Huddleston. The former concludes her letter thus:

If you have any of the Philtre to spare, there is nothing I can think of I should like much better!

Believe me, dear Mr. J. W. W.,
Yours sincerely,
CONSTANCE WESTMINSTER.

---

The initials had reference to John Wellington Wells, the part in *The Sorcerer* I was playing at the time.

I had sent Lady Diana the name of a professional spiritualist, and here is an extract from her reply:

Thank you so much for writing to E——. I am all for a medium who stands no nonsense with the spirits, but has them up there and then. I fear W—— lets his ghosties give themselves airs, as both "Petre" and also "John King" have always thrown me over. Who was John King? . . .

Yours very sincerely,
DI. HUDDLESTON.

---

Letters of invitation follow from Frank Holl, R.A., George du Maurier, Nita Gäetana (Mrs. Moncrieff), Kate Field, and Earls of Fife and Wharncliffe. Then comes a letter from F. C. Burnand, respecting my proposer for the Beefsteak Club. He suggested Sir Arthur Sullivan;

but eventually Corney Grain proposed me. I think Frank Burnand is the most amusing man to meet. He is brimful of good humour. He will fire off joke after joke, and chaff you out of your life if he gets a chance. His chaff is always good-tempered. No one minds being chaffed by Burnand. I will not sing a song when he is in the room if I can possibly help it. He will sit in front of me at the piano, and either stare with a pained and puzzled look during my comic song, or he will laugh in the wrong places, or, what is worse still, take out his pocket-handkerchief and weep.

A short time ago we were dining at Mrs. Lovett Cameron's, and were seated on either side of her. Throughout the dinner I had purposely been making some rude observations respecting the dishes, with which Mrs. Cameron was immensely amused. Eventually a "sweet" was handed round, consisting of little hard cakes of something resembling dark-brown toffee or hardbake, with cream piled on. Mrs. Cameron said to me, "You must not pass this dish—*do* have some." I replied, "Well, I won't have any of the cream—only some of the *glue*," which the sweet certainly resembled. Burnand promptly replied, "Oh, are you going to *stick* here all night?"

Burnand's parties are to be envied, and not forgotten. At one of his evening entertainments in Russell Square, he suggested we should get up a "bogus" band. I fell in with his idea at once, and it was left to me to arrange. I decided upon the overture to *Zampa*; and, to give a semblance of reality to the performance, arranged with Mr. Charles Reddie to preside at the piano; and, chaos or no chaos, he was to go steadily on. Frederic H. Cowen was the violoncello; the first violins were played by Mr. Samuel Heilbut, a capital amateur violinist, and by my brother, who was nearly as good. I played second violin, and was simply awful. Rutland Barrington played the piccolo; but as he could only play in one key, which, unfortunately, was *not* the one we were playing, the effect can be imagined. Last, but not least, Corney Grain conducted.

The time arrived for the performance, and the music-stands were placed in a circle in the crowded drawing-room; and, in order that there should be no jumble at the commencement, we decided to take the overture at exactly half its proper time.

I shall never forget the surprised look on the faces of Sir Julius Benedict and Mr. W. G. Cusins when we began. There was no idea, at first, it was a joke. We played the next *andante* movement with sublime expression and perfectly correctly, with the exception of Barrington's piccolo, which was here more terribly conspicuous than before. This was rendered all the more ridiculous by the sweet, satisfied smile which Grain was assuming, after the fashion of an affected conductor.

The audience began to suspect something was up; but their suspicions were soon set at rest when the subsequent quick movement arrived. Reddie played on, and Heilbut stuck to it. Fred. Cowen, Weedon Grossmith, and myself put down our instruments and stared up at the ceiling, as if we had a few bars' rest. Barrington played a tune of his own; and Grain, in an excited manner and in the German tongue, demanded him to desist. Barrington, who also speaks German, retaliated.

This German row was most natural and funny, and created roars of laughter. J. L. Toole, who was in the audience, and who did not see why he should not join in, forced his way through the people and seized hold of Weedon's old Italian violin, and was about to bang it on the back of a chair. Weedon had a genuine fight to recover his fiddle, and had to remind Toole that it was not one of his own "properties." Reddie and Heilbut still seriously stuck to the piano and violin. Grain then bullied me for not playing. A general altercation ensued; and as the final chords of the shortened overture were played, Grain seized me up under his arm, as if I had been a brown-paper parcel, and marched out of the room with me.

After supper there was an extemporised Christmas Pantomime, in which Grain, Arthur Cecil, Fred. Leslie, Chas. Colnaghi, William Yardley, the brothers Grossmith, and Mrs. Cecil Clay (Miss Rosina Vokes) took part. It was great fun for audience and performers, and Miss Vokes was excellent. At the final tableau, Fred. Leslie and myself struck two matches to represent coloured fire. I daresay all this seems silly; but I have seen many very serious people silly after a jolly supper with jolly people, so I hope some allowance will be made for the Society Clown.

A little pencil sketch, by W. S. Gilbert, comes next in my book; "Bab" is an excellent draughtsman, as everyone knows. Next on the list are Annie Thomas (Mrs. Pender Cudlip) and Florence Marryat. The latter often signed herself "The Ship," because one of the Birmingham papers, speaking of the "Entre Nous" entertainment, described her as "of pleasant appearance, with bright, frank features, somewhat massively moulded, unaffected manners, and with a carriage reminding one of the stately motion of one of those noble vessels of which the glorious old Captain loved to write." The same paper, continuing, observes: "In the second costume recital of 'Joan of Arc in prison,' she appeared in the usual grey tunic and with massive manacles on her waist; Mr. Grossmith, sitting at the piano as a sort of mute but comical gaoler, ready to accompany her in a musical scéna at the end."

I have before said that Arthur Cecil took a kind interest in me, and favoured me with many a valuable hint. I therefore print a letter of his (dated 1878, when I knew him only slightly) in full, with the assurance, from experience, that jealousy in the theatrical profession is the exception and not the rule:

Beefsteak Club,
King William Street,
Strand, W.C.

My dear Grossmith,—I am so delighted to hear you "obliged again" on Wednesday, at Grosvenor House, after I left.

I was most anxious that you should be at your best before the Prince and Princess, and only regretted I could not stop to suggest the things that I consider your happiest efforts. I am sure "The Muddle Puddle Porter" must have been all right.

Yours ever,

Arthur C. Blunt.

---

It was a charity concert, and I may incidentally remark that I had to appear early in the programme, and when my turn came their Royal Highnesses had not arrived. Arthur Cecil, who was announced later on, said: "The Prince and Princess have heard my song, so you take my place."

The above voluntary suggestion on his part needs no comment.

This letter is followed by ordinary letters from Irving, Toole, A. W. Pinero, Countess of Charlemont (the late), Viscountess Combermere, Herbert Herkomer, A.R.A., Earls of Londesborough and Dunraven, Mrs. Charlie Mathews, Mrs. Kendal, the Hon. Lewis Wingfield, Emily Faithful, and Kate Terry (Mrs. Arthur Lewis). Then comes a letter from Thomas Thorne, which is interesting because it is an invitation to dine with him to celebrate the thousandth night of *Our Boys*. Then follow Robert Reece (he persuaded me to set to music one of his songs, "A Peculiar Man," which he need not have done, for he is a most excellent musician himself), John Oxenford (dated 1868—a birthday congratulation), J. Ashby Sterry (who always addresses me "dear young Jaärge"), R. Corney Grain, Herman Vezin, Lord Otho Fitzgerald, and Viscountess

Mandeville. The letter from Lady Mandeville, referring to some of my songs, is amusing—an extract from which I give:

Thanks a thousand times for the songs, which were delightful. We tried them all last night and I am sure some of the neighbours wished us at the North Pole. . . . I have sent to America for a charming pathetic song for you; the last line is " Let me hit my little brother before I die."

A letter from J. B. Buckstone, giving me permission to play Paul Pry *(en amateur)*; a most amusing letter from Howard Paul, describing his futile attempt to learn " The Muddle Puddle Porter " while " going up and down the Lake of Lucerne, under the shadow of the Rigi, and within sight of the historical Tell's Platte;" a most flattering letter from Sir Julius Benedict, which modesty, &c., will not permit of my reproducing; Jacques Blumenthal (he simply had "a message to send me" inviting me to dine) and Henry J. Byron. I knew Byron when I was a boy, and I loved him because he was not above playing cricket with me on the sands at the seaside, when I was in trousers, or rather knickerbockers, which they resembled through my having outgrown them. In 1878 I wanted to purchase some clever words of his with a refrain, " Yeo, heave ho." He wrote back from the Haymarket Theatre:

Dear George,—I wrote to you, saying you might have the song gratis, and posted the letter to J. S. Clarke instead of you.

Yours ever sincerely,

H. J. BYRON.

Everybody knows Byron was about the best punster existing. He was also the worst. I heard him make this observation at Margate: "I don't like *cock*roaches because they '*en*-croaches."

Then come Arthur à Beckett, Countesses of Wharncliffe and Bantry, S. B. Bancroft, Lionel Brough, Viscounts Hardinge and Baring; a charming letter from Clement Scott, asking me for a contribution to a collection of theatrical stories; Sir Algernon Borthwick, Duke of Beaufort, Earl of Hardwicke, and Mrs. Keeley. The letter (dated 1882) from the latter lady, I value most highly, of course:

10 Pelham Crescent, S.W.

Dear Mr. Grossmith,—I was at the Savoy on Thursday evening with Miss Swanborough, and delighted we were with the performance. Trusting yourself and Madame are well, and with kind regards,

Ever yours sincerely,<br>MARY ANNE KEELEY.

---

17 Finchley New Road,<br>*Thursday*.

Dear Mr. Grossmith,—I am not going to use any flourishing phrases, but simply ask you if you would be so extremely good as to appear in the concert I arrange for the poor exiles at Walmer. It is to be on the 15th or 18th of this month, in the house of Lord Denbigh. I am going to play a little French piece with M. Berton, and I asked some artists to play and sing. I hope you will frankly tell me if you can do it or not, as I certainly should not like you to put yourself to any inconvenience for my sake. I know how busy you are, and it is a great impudence on my part to give you some more work. With many kind regards,

    I remain, always sincerely yours,
        HELENA MODJESKA.

"Next, please," as Mr. T. Thorne would say, as Partridge.

H.S.H. the Duke of Teck, Countess of Kenmare, James Albery (author of *The Two Roses*), Henry Labouchere, Miss E. Braddon, Joseph Hatton (a very old and esteemed friend of mine) and Professor Pepper.

The following is interesting to me, coming, as it does, from the most successful entertainer of his day. His songs, "A Life on the Ocean Wave," "Cheer, Boys, Cheer," "The Ivy Green," "The Ship on Fire," etc., will be ever remembered:

    Hanover Square Club,
     *Nov. 22nd*, 1883.

My dear Grossmith,—Many thanks for your kind letter. I leave for Boulogne to-morrow (Friday), or I should be only too glad to avail myself of your generous offer. I have been for years one of the warmest admirers of the great talent you possess; and all I can say is, that if you want to confer a favour on me, you will, without hesitation, jump on board the Boulogne boat, and, after two hours of "a life on the ocean wave," come direct to the Hotel du Nord, where I reside, and where you shall have a good dinner, a glorious weed, a first-class bottle of Château Margaux, a shake-down, and a sincere warm welcome from your old friend,   HENRY RUSSELL.

Grand Hotel, Stockholm,
*June* 13*th*, 1882.

Dear Grossmith,—I have just remembered you have received no reply to your invite for the "small and early." . . . We left London on the 6th, and since then have visited Hamburg and Copenhagen. To-night we start for Christiania on our way to the North Cape. Should any friends ask my address, tell them for the next three weeks, " Arctic Ocean."

Kind regards from Mrs. and self to Mrs. G. and self.

Yours sincerely,
Edward Terry.

---

The following is from Nellie Farren:

Gaiety Theatre, Strand,
*Friday.*

Dear George,—Will you repeat yesterday's performance on the 23rd of this month for your old friend,

Nell.

---

Alfred Scott Gatty, Hamilton Aïdé, Duke of Abercorn, Earl of Onslow, William J. Florence (the popular American comedian), John Hare, W. Kuhé, W. Maybrick (his "Nancy Lee" still haunts me), Chas. Wyndham, W. J. Hill, Oscar Wilde, and J. McNiel Whistler, from whose epistle I give an extract:

" Je tu savois brave—mais je ne tu savois pas plus brave que moy ! "

Ton roy, Henri.

Which means, my dear Bunthorne, that " I knew you amazing !—but I did not know you more amazing than I " !

                      Thine

Then appears the well-known " butterfly " signature.

---

Madam Dolby, Madam Liebhart, Viscountess Folkestone, Lady Coutts Lindsay (whose charming collections of people at the Grosvenor Gallery some years ago will not be easily forgotten), Beatty Kingston, Frederick Boyle, Manville Fenn, Lady Chas. Beresford, Marchioness of Ormond, Lady Chesham, G. H. Boughton, A.R.A., Pro. Ray Lankester, Sir Coutts Lindsay, Earl and Countess of Donoughmore. Her ladyship writes :

. . . I am afraid we cannot go to London this season. There is an idea that digging turnips at Knocklofty would be a pleasing change. I should not mind the turnips if kind friends would come and help dig them. Have you and Mrs. Grossmith any sharp spuds, and would you like to race me in a drill ? (I don't know if turnips are planted in drills—potatoes are.) Are you afraid of the sea ? It's not very rough, and your chicks could play and fight with mine all day, and we would have a good time somehow.

---

Mrs. Alfred Wigan, Carlotta Leclercq, Viscountess Pollington, Harry Furniss, E. Willard, Sir Morell Mackenzie, Duchess of Abercorn (a kind letter referring to my severe illness in Jan., 1887), Harry Payne (certainly the best clown in my time), Rutland Barrington, Fred. Leslie, Meyer Lutz, Earl of Clarendon.

Pro. Hubert Herkomer, A.R.A., writes, in reply to my enquiry whether he was busy:

I am now at work on my thirty-first portrait this year—which does not count water-colour subjects. Can't you spend a Sunday with me?

---

Milton Wellings, Lord Hay of Kinfauns, Arthur Stirling.

*July 15th*, 1887.

Dear Grossmith,—We are looking forward with very great pleasure to lunching with you next Monday.

My duty to your wife.

Yours ever,

DOUGLAS STRAIGHT.

---

11 Melbury Road, W.
*20th April*, 1887.

My dear Grossmith,—No congratulations I have received have given me more pleasure than those coming from old friends, and among them I was gratified to have yours; for we have known each other a long time, and I believe with corresponding regard. Accept my very best thanks for your nice letter; and with best wishes for yourself and your wife,

I am, sincerely yours,

LUKE FILDES.

Sir Edward Sieveking, Baroness Burdett Coutts (a kind invitation for my wife and myself to see the Jubilee procession), Paul Rajon (the French etcher), E. Gibert (whom the *Daily Telegraph* flattered me by designating the French Grossmith).

The following, from Hamilton Clarke, had reference to a small theatre work of mine which I had to score for an exceedingly limited orchestra:

Dear George,—Yardley tells me to send you a list of the band at —— theatre.

I regret to say that, owing to the fact that the accommodation for the musicians is about the dimensions of a third-class railway compartment (I believe the trombone-player has to play lying down), the "orchestra" is limited to the following list: . . . No chance of the slightest delicacy or fancy! Only plain, straightforward English slogging.

Long live the cornet and side-drum—Briton's boast!
Yours sincerely,
Hamilton Clarke.

---

33 Longridge Road,
Earl's Court,
*December 20th.*

Dear George,—£3, if you don't mind; and I am so sorry for the poor lady. I've just come back from Paris, and your letter had been sent there and back here after me, or you would have heard from me before. Hope you are very well. With love to you both,
Yours ever,
Ellen Terry.

I'm having a lovely Christmas holiday.

Percy Fitzgerald (I shall naturally look forward to his *Chronicles of Bow Street* with special interest), Emily Lovett Cameron, Joseph Hollman, Duchess of Westminster (the present), H. S. Marks, R.A., Arthur Roberts, C. D. Marius, Wilford Morgan, George Giddens, Dr. Anderson Critchett, Bottesini, H.S.H. Prince Leiningen, Sir Frederick Leighton, P.R.A.

White Lodge,
Richmond Park,
*January 7th.*

Dear Mr. Grossmith,—I thank you for sending me your photos; it was a very kind thought of you. I trust Ko-Ko and yourself to be in the best of spirits. I must go to the Savoy again, and I hope you will from thence proceed with me to the Bachelor's and have some supper.

Yours sincerely,
TECK.

33 Untere Promenade,
Homburg,
*Saturday.*

Dear Grossmith,—The Prince of Wales hopes that Mrs. Grossmith and you will dine with him at the Kinsaal on Monday evening, at 7.15.

Yours truly,
H. TYRWHITT-WILSON.

I had promised to write David James a song for *Little Jack Sheppard*, at the Gaiety,—a promise which I failed to keep. I had a good "intention," but not an "idea." The reward for my failure was this amusing letter:

> 14 Buckingham Street,
> Adelphi,
> *May* 2*nd*, 1886.
>
> Dear Grossmith,—The *song* you wrote for me for Blueskin goes IMMENSELY every night, and everybody is asking who is the *author* and *composer*. Now, as you cannot come and bow your acknowledgments at *night*, you might as well come and do so in the *morning;* and what better morning than Thursday, the 20th of May, at my *matinée* benefit at the Gaiety? I want all my old pals to be there. . . . Like a good boy, come and sing and play, and very much oblige
>
> Your old " partic.,"
> DAVID JAMES.

---

A. Goring Thomas, Percy Reeve, Sir Percy Shelley, Fred. Barnard (with humorous sketch), John T. Bedford (author of " Robert," in *Punch*).

> Lyceum Theatre,
> 16*th February*, 1887.
>
> Dear Grossmith,—Greeting! Right hearty congratulations on your recovery and reappearance this evening.
>
> Sincerely yours,
> H. IRVING.

---

A letter from Lady Freake reminds me of (to me) a memorable performance at Cromwell

House. The musical triumviretta, *Cox and Box*, formed part of the programme:

| | |
|---|---|
| Box ... ... ... ... ... ... | Mr. ARTHUR CECIL. |
| Cox ... ... ... ... ... ... | Mr. GEORGE GROSSMITH. |
| Serjeant Bouncer... ... ... | Mr. CORNEY GRAIN. |

| | |
|---|---|
| *Piano* ... ... ... | Mr. ALFRED CELLIER. |
| *Harmonium* ... ... | Sir ARTHUR SULLIVAN. |

I remember seeing at this entertainment the Dowager Countess of Waldegrave, who was the daughter of John Braham, the celebrated singer. But what most impressed me was an incident at the first rehearsal. Cecil, Grain, and I were under the impression that we had the well-fitted little theatre to ourselves; but suddenly two elderly and very prim ladies came and sat in the front row and watched us. There is nothing so disconcerting to actors as to be watched at the preliminary rehearsal. I cannot bear it even at the dress rehearsal. In the present instance we grumbled to ourselves and delayed commencing, hoping the two ladies would take the hint and depart. No such luck. One of them, the mother of an exceedingly clever amateur who has played *Cox and Box* all his life (I believe he was born playing it), suddenly said, in a loud voice:

"Why don't they begin? Don't they know what to do? I wish Johnnie were here; he could show them at once."

Royal Princess's Theatre,
*March 23rd, 1886.*

Dear Grossmith,—I know one "little piece" only, "Gone with a handsomer man." If that will do, I am ready to help you; unless it should be

the date on which *Clito* is produced. I expect to play it earlier than that. Kind regards.
Faithfully yours,
WILSON BARRETT.

---

Miss Hope Glen, Isidore de Lara, Wilhelm Ganz, Linley Sambourne, Charles Warner, Fred. H. Cowen, E. W. Royce, Miss Fortescue (informing me of the breaking off of the engagement between herself and Lord Garmoyle, now Earl Cairns), John Clayton, Lady Mildred Denison, Lady William Lennox, Lady Ventry, Lady Ardilaun, M. Rivière, Sir John Bennett, Madame Lemmens-Sherrington.

I am frequently asked, when singing professionally in private houses, if I am friendly with Mr. Corney Grain. Here is an extract from one of his letters. I had been suffering from sore throat, and could not fulfil a certain engagement, and he kindly sang in my stead. In return, I sent him a small souvenir in the shape of a " Tantalus."

Dear George,—Thank you very much for your very handsome—and, moreover, very useful—present. It shall be entirely at your service from March 21st till the 6th April, when I hope, barring accidents, to be at The Willows, Datchet, where you have, not a general, but a particular invitation during that period.

---

Another of his letters terminates thus :
Then farewell my trim-built wherry.
From that sheer hulk,
R. CORNEY GRAIN.

Countess of Bective, Marshall P. Wilder (the American humorist), Gordon Thomson, Sir John Millais, John Hollingshead, Earl of Hopetoun.

At a party at Sir Arthur Sullivan's one evening, I was asked to sing the Lord Chancellor's enormous patter song. I could not remember it; so Lord Hopetoun, himself a most excellent humorous singer, volunteered to prompt me. The effect was most ludicrous; for Lord Hopetoun had really to sing quickly the whole of the song about one bar ahead of me. After this, Sir Arthur sat at the piano, and Lord Hopetoun and myself arrayed ourselves in a few antimacassars and performed a graceful ballet; that is to say, as graceful as the circumstances would permit.

A kind letter from my old friend, Alfred Cellier, respecting the death of my father, reminds me of another evening at Sir Arthur Sullivan's. We had been previously to a dinner-party and subsequent reception at Lady Sebright's, where I was introduced to Mrs. Langtry—it being, I believe, her first introduction to London Society.

Subsequently, Sullivan persuaded Cellier, Arthur Cecil, and myself, and I fancy a few others, including Archibald Stuart Wortley, to return to his rooms at 9 Albert Mansions, where the gifted composer was then residing. We stayed very late—much later than I would dare stay up now. I left with Alfred Cellier, and he asked me if I could drop him in Park Lane, as he had another party to go to. There was every excuse for my being astonished, considering it was half-past four in the morning and the beautiful daylight had long since appeared. I acquiesced, and the next day asked Cellier if he did not find that everybody had gone.

"No, indeed," replied Cellier; "in fact, I was the *first arrival*."

Rather an early card party!

Speaking of Mrs. Langtry, recalls to my mind a curious incident affecting both of us. I was asked to a musical party in Prince's Gardens, and proceeded there after my work at the theatre. On arriving in the locality, and seeing the awning out, and the usual line of footmen, and the will-o'-the-wisp linkman, I shouted to the cabman, who was passing the door, to stop. I gave up my coat and walked into the drawing-room, being announced in the usual way. I found, however, that a ball was in full swing. I could not discover my host or hostess, although I met many people I knew. I soon ascertained that I had come to the wrong house, and, instead of being at Mrs. G——'s musical party, was at Sir William D——'s ball. I slipped downstairs—having ex-explained the matter to a friend of Sir William's—got my coat, and went to Mrs. G——'s, which was a few doors off. As I was proceeding upstairs I met Mrs. Langtry coming down, and she said:

"Oh, Mr. Grossmith, I've made *such* a mistake! I've come to the wrong house. I ought to be at the ball at Sir William D——'s. I couldn't understand how it was there was singing and no dancing upstairs, and have only just discovered my mistake."

I replied, "You may be comforted; I have

been to Sir William D——'s by mistake, when I ought to have been here."

Lady Greville, Madame de Fonblanque, Brindley Richards, Henry S. Neville (asking me to play " Paul Pry " at the Crystal Palace), Earl of Desart, who, in kindly sending me an invitation, described the whereabouts of his house thus :

> "There's a place called Victoria Lodge,
> It lies in Victoria Street ;
> To find it, I'll tell you the dodge—
> Ask ev'ry policeman you meet."

H. Beerbohm Tree, Countess of Wilton, Miss Millward, Dr. Louis Engel, H. Bracy, Kate Vaughan.

Marlborough House,
Pall Mall, S.W.,
*June* 30th, 1885.

Dear Mr. Grossmith,—By direction of the Prince and Princess of Wales, I send you the accompanying pin, which their Royal Highnesses hope you will accept as a small souvenir of your visit to Marlborough House on the evening of the 14th inst.

Believe me, yours truly,
———   D. M. Probyn.

Court Theatre,
Sloane Square, S.W.,
*March* 30th.

My dear George,—Many thanks for your kind letter. The play, so far, promises to exceed *The Magistrate*.

Yours truly,
John Clayton.

> 145 Harley Street, W.,

Dear Mr. Grossmith,—I have been asked by people right and left; but put my name down, and if I can recite—I will.

> Yours faithfully,
> MADGE KENDAL.

---

> 156 Cambridge Street,
> Warwick Square, S.W.

My dear Grossmith,—One line to say "Thank you;" another from my mother to repeat the "Thank you." The two joined make the words bear their fullest measure of truth, and your kindness is very pleasant to

> Yours sincerely,
> CLIFFORD HARRISON.

---

Dear Mr. Grossmith,—I will (D.V.) be there on the 4th. Many thanks.

> Yours ever truly,
> M. E. BANCROFT.

---

> 46 Russell Square,
> *March 19th*, 1884.

Dear Gee Gee ("I've spotted you"),—You'd do much more good if you'd just leave *Cox and Box* alone, and stick to writing what I ask you to. I chuckled over this week's *Very Trying*, No. VIII. Capital. I've written to Committee, and told 'em Weedon is a *much better* fellow than you are. *Ergo*, if they like *you*, they'll elect Weedon; if they *don't* like you, *still* they'll elect Weedon.

> Q.E.D.
> Yours ever,
> F. C. BURNAND.

6 Hill Street,
24*th May*, 1884.

Dear Mr. Grossmith,—I am very much obliged to you for your note and the photos sent with it. My daughter will write her own thanks for your note addressed to her.

I take the liberty of sending you one of my photographs in return for those you have so kindly sent me.

With many thanks,
I remain,
Very truly yours,
WOLSELEY.

---

*May* 14*th*.

My dear Grossmith,—I am desired by the Duke of Albany to invite Mrs. Grossmith and yourself to lunch at Claremont, on Friday next, before the concert. A train leaves Waterloo for Esher at 12.15, by which I hope you will come. Please send a line in reply to the Comptroller of the Household, Claremont, Esher; and

Believe me,
Yours very sincerely,
ALEC YORKE.

---

Sainte Croix,
Upper East Sheen,
Mortlake,
*June* 13*th*, 1887.

My dear George Grossmith,—I hope there is no doubt about you and your wife giving us the pleasure of sharing our housewarming on the 6th prox.; for, in addition to the gratification of having you both with us, I want you to volunteer a song on the occasion. . . . You mustn't ridicule the idea of my giving a housewarming at my time of life, for on the 27th inst. I shall have achieved my 70th year; but the meeting of old friends under a new roof will be a cheery event to look back upon by an aged pilgrim who is starting a new family home in his 71st year.

With kindest regards to Mrs. Grossmith,

Believe me,
My dear George Grossmith,
Faithfully yours,
T. GERMAN REED.

---

The following is from the once famous clown, the legitimate successor to Grimaldi, with whom he played:

51 Upper Lewes Road,
Brighton,
*October 8th*, 1885.

My dear Mr. Grossmith,—Yours to hand. Many thanks for the kind epistle respecting my birthday and health. I should like to have seen you. Pray give me a call next time you visit Brighton. God bless my dear, kind, good old friend, John L. Toole. Excuse my being brief. Shakespeare says, "Let those who play your clowns, speak no more than is put down for them."

So I remain,
Very faithfully yours,
TOM MATTHEWS.

Eighty years of age October 17th, 1885.
Excuse all mistakes, my sight is bad.

He does not show it in his letter; for he had sketched, in coloured crayons, a tiny representation of himself in the motley—head and shoulders.

Sir Rivers Wilson, Eric Lewis, Lord Garmoyle (now Earl Cairns), Frank Miles, Herman Merivale, Kyrle Bellew, Jules Lasserre, Brandon Thomas, Alfred German Reed, Lady Fanny Fitzwygram, Mrs. Arthur Stirling, Alice Barnett (Lady Jane in *Patience*), Leonora Braham, Jessie Bond, Jenny Lee (Jo), Carlotta Addison, Alfred Scott Gatty, Countess of Londesborough (asking me to sit with his lordship and "cheer him up" at the time of his dreadful accident), Lady Dorothy Nevill.

Everybody knows that Lady Dorothy Nevill gives very charming luncheon parties, their chief characteristic being the odd assortment of celebrities. On one of these occasions the announcement of the guests, who, somehow or other, arrived in strange couples, was especially amusing. The servant threw open the drawing-room doors, and announced "Lord Pembroke and Mr. George Grossmith." As I am only five-feet-five in height and comic in appearance, and his lordship is six-feet-six and rather serious, it is not to be wondered at that those already assembled indulged in a titter. The next announcement by the servant was "The Earl of Wharncliffe and Mr. Justin McCarthy." For political reasons alone, this was amusing. Then came "The Duke of Wellington and Mr. Corney Grain." I do not know why, but this sounded very funny. It is only fair to Lady Dorothy to state that these are not "surprise" parties. Her guests are always informed whom they are to meet.

The following letter is *àpropos* of my *début* at the Opéra Comique:

> The Green Room,
> 10 Adelphi Terrace, W.C.,
> *December* 10*th*, 1877.
>
> Dear George,—Let me congratulate you very heartily on your success. I read with very great pleasure the good notices about you. I shall hope to *hear* you soon; because when at "The Globe" I shall cut a hole in the wall, and hope to listen to the charming music whilst I'm going through my own performance.
>
> With kind regards to your wife and self, and all good wishes for your continued success in your new arena,
>
> I am,
> Yours sincerely,
> J. L. TOOLE.

Besides being a very old and privileged friend of the famous and popular comedian, I have had the pleasure of being associated with him in business, having composed the music for *Mr. Guffin's Elopement* and *The Great Tay-kins*, written by Arthur Law, and produced at Toole's theatre.

Toole is fond of stories about other people. Here is one about him. Not being a musician, and not being a quick study, it becomes no easy task to drum a song, or especially duet, into his head. In *The Great Tay-kins* there was a "one-line-each" duet between him and Mr. E. D. Ward. I could not get Toole to get the rhythm right. He kept saying it was all right, but it was not. This is what it ought to have been:

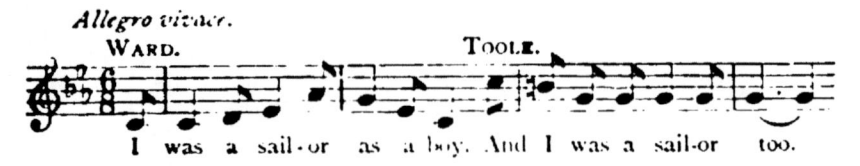

[Musical notation: Allegro vivace. WARD / TOOLE. "I was a sail-or as a boy. And I was a sail-or too."]

This is how Toole first got it:

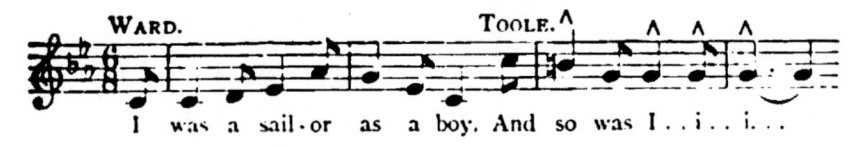

[Musical notation: WARD / TOOLE. "I was a sail-or as a boy. And so was I..i..i..."]

After a dozen rehearsals of these few bars, he got it thus:

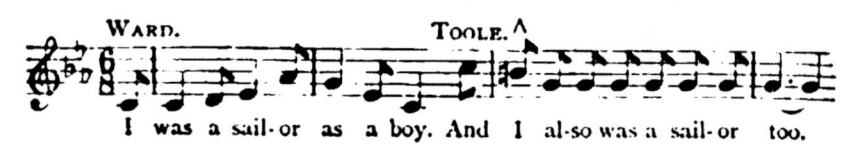

[Musical notation: WARD / TOOLE. "I was a sail-or as a boy. And I al-so was a sail-or too."]

The company were in roars of laughter; but Toole struggled on perfectly seriously until he got it. He was then as pleased as Punch, and insisted on my lunching with him, an invitation I was not likely to refuse.

The following is from Sir Algernon Borthwick, who was my proposer for the Garrick Club:

*Morning Post,*
*February 17th, 1883.*

Dear Grossmith,—You were elected this afternoon, not only unanimously, but with warmest expressions of welcome and goodwill. I never saw so cordial and sympathetic an election.

Sincerely yours,
ALGERNON BORTHWICK.

*March* 29*th*, 1882.

My dear Grossmith,—If you are not too tired, and have no better engagement, will you come up and see my "show"—all portraits (Chamber of Horrors)—before they go to the R.A. on Friday evening? The usual business—not dress.

Yours sincerely,<br>FRANK HOLL.

---

*From* Mrs. JOHN WOOD.

23 Gordon Square, W.C.,<br>*July* 10*th*, Midnight.

My dear George,—I cannot go to rest to-night without thanking you really and truly for your invaluable help this afternoon, and for the very graceful courtesy you have shown through the entire affair. I can only say if at any time I can do anything for you, you will confer a favour on me by asking it. Your dear little wife cheered me by saying she and everybody were very pleased with us, and I don't think she would have said so if she hadn't meant it. So good-night to you both, and God bless you.

Your faithful friend,<br>MATILDA WOOD.

---

The following, from George M. du Maurier, the incomparable *Punch* artist, has reference to the death of "Chang," the enormous dog which he possessed, and which he so often immortalised on the pages of the above periodical:

New Grove House,
Hampstead Heath.

We are all (especially I) much touched by your kind note about poor old "Chang," whom we miss very much. Although his death was expected, it was very painful when it came, more so than I should have thought possible in the case of an animal. His bones have gone to the museum of the College of Surgeons, and his skin is coming back to me. He was so big that, having no groom or manservant to look after him, I had to be his slave, and nothing is so attaching as voluntary slavery; so that I cannot yet rejoice in my new-found liberty. Please thank your wife for me for her kind feeling.

---

12 The Terrace,
Kennington Park, S.E.,
*October 1st, 1885.*

Dear Grossmith,—On the 29th inst. I make my last appeal to the public, and on that occasion I want all the friendly support I can obtain. May I ask the favour of your vocal assistance? If agreeable and convenient, the programme will be complete.

Yours faithfully,
WM. CRESWICK.

---

Marlborough House,
*May 16th, 1888.*

Dear Mr. Grossmith,—The Princess has desired me to thank you for so kindly sending her that prettily-bound collection of your songs. H.R.H. is delighted to have it, and will value and prize the book extremely.

Believe me, yours truly,<br>
CHARLOTTE KNOLLYS.

---

I naturally conclude "my little list" with letters from Gilbert and Sullivan, to whom I shall ever feel grateful for their many kindnesses and the opportunities they have offered me of more or less distinguishing myself:

19 Harrington Gardens,<br>
South Kensington,<br>
24th February, 1884.

My dear Grossmith,—Carte tells me you had made some engagement for to-morrow afternoon. If so, pray don't trouble to come down to the theatre, as I know *your* business is all right. But some of the others have become slack, and want bracing up.

Yours faithfully,<br>
W. S. GILBERT.

During my dangerous illness, Mr. Gilbert never failed a day to come up and enquire after me. He also came down to Brighton with D'Oyly Carte, and kept me in roars of laughter the whole time. This was one of the bright days during an anxious time. But to see Gilbert at his best, is to see him at one of his juvenile parties. Though he has no children of his own, he loves them, and there is nothing he would not do to please them. I was never so astonished as when on one occasion he put off some of his own friends to come with Mrs. Gilbert to a juvenile party at my own house.

The following had reference to a mock melodrama, written by myself, which Barrington, my brother, and I were to act at Sir Arthur's on an occasion when he was entertaining the Prince of Wales, the Duke of Edinburgh, and other distinguished guests:

1 Queen's Mansions,<br>Victoria Street, S.W.

Dear Grossmith,—Are you down in this neighbourhood to-morrow any time? If so, we might run through the "melos" here, or I could meet you in town (Chappell's) at 3.30. Send me a wire early, please.

I hope Mrs. Grossmith will come; and, furthermore, that she understands that I shall never send her a separate invitation, as I shall always be delighted to see her whenever you come. It does not, of course, follow that I shall be delighted to see *you* whenever *she* comes.

Yours sincerely,<br>ARTHUR SULLIVAN.

Hotel de Paris,<br>Monte Carlo,<br>28th February, 1887.

Dear G. G.,—The earthquake knocked me about so much mentally, that I could not write sooner to you to say how glad I am that you are all right again—for both our sakes. Don't get ill again, but take care of yourself. We are all calm again here, but we had a nasty time of it. I think the suspense afterwards was worse than the shock itself. . . .

Yours sincerely,<br>ARTHUR SULLIVAN.

The following is an instance of the good feeling that has always existed between the authors and actors:

> 1 Queen's Mansions,
> Victoria Street, S.W.,
> 15th *January*, 1884.
>
> My dear Grossmith,—Many thanks for your very kind letter. It is pleasant to be thought of when one is ill; and it is also pleasant to know that one's works are in the hands, not only of artists, but of *friends* like yourself, who bring something more than a mere professional interest to bear on their work. I have had a very sharp and severe attack; but, fortunately, a short one. I have been out three times for a drive, and to-day go into the country till Friday. My kind remembrances to Mrs. Grossmith.
>
> Yours sincerely,
> ARTHUR SULLIVAN.

On second thoughts, I will conclude with a letter from myself to the purchasers of *A Society Clown*:

Dear Readers,—If I have succeeded in amusing or interesting you, I shall feel myself more than repaid for my trouble. If I have bored or disappointed you, I beg to offer my apologies; for it was not my intention to do so.

Your grateful and obedient Servant,
GEORGE GROSSMITH.

28 Dorset Square,
*July*, 1888.

FINIS.